God's Design for the
Highly Healthy
Child

Resources by Dr. Walt Larimore

Bryson City Seasons

Bryson City Tales

Alternative Medicine: The Christian Handbook
(coauthored with Dónal O'Mathúna)

God's Design for the Highly Healthy Person
(with Traci Mullins)

God's Design for the Highly Healthy Child
(with Stephen and Amanda Sorenson)

God's Design for the Highly Healthy Teen
(with Mike Yorkey)

Why ADHD Doesn't Mean Disaster
(coauthored with Dennis Swanberg and Diane Passno)

Lintball Leo's Not-So-Stupid Questions About Your Body
(with John Riddle, illustrated by Mike Phillips)

Going Public with Your Faith: Becoming a Spiritual Influence at Work
(coauthored with William Carr Peel)

Going Public with Your Faith: Becoming a Spiritual Influence at Work
audio
(coauthored with William Carr Peel)

Going Public with Your Faith: Becoming a Spiritual Influence at Work
Zondervan *Groupware*™ curriculum
(coauthored with William Carr Peel, with Stephen
and Amanda Sorenson)

God's Design *for the*
Highly Healthy Child

Formerly titled *The Highly Healthy Child*

Walt Larimore, M.D.

WITH STEPHEN & AMANDA SORENSON

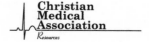

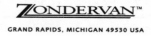

GRAND RAPIDS, MICHIGAN 49530 USA

We want to hear from you. Please send your comments about this
book to us in care of zreview@zondervan.com. Thank you.

ZONDERVAN™

God's Design for the Highly Healthy Child
Copyright © 2004 by Walt Larimore

Requests for information should be addressed to:
Zondervan, *Grand Rapids, Michigan 49530*

Library of Congress Cataloging-in-Publication Data

Larimore, Walter L.
  [Highly healthy child]
  God's design for the highly healthy child / Walt Larimore, with Stephen and Amanda
  Sorenson—
  1st. ed.
       p. cm.
     "Formerly titled: The highly healthy child."
     Includes bibliographical references and index.
     ISBN 0-310-26283-6 (softcover)
     1. Children—Health and hygiene   2. Children—Diseases—Prevention.
  3. Child development.   I. Sorenson, Stephen   II. Sorenson, Amanda, 1953–   III. Title.
  RJ101 .L37 2004b
  649'.1—dc22
                                                                    2004019429

Interior design by Michelle Espinoza

Printed in the United States of America

---

04 05 06 07 08 09 10 /❖ DCI/ 10 9 8 7 6 5 4 3 2 1

To Kate and Scott—
not only are you precious gifts to your mom and me,
you are indeed highly healthy.

Contents

Foreword

At times guesswork can be fun. For example,

- in which sport do neither the spectators nor the participants know the score of the leader until the contest ends?
- which fruit has its seeds on the outside?
- what are the only three words in standard English that begin with the letters "dw" (all three are commonly used)?
- which famous North American landmark is constantly moving *backward*?

Taking a guess when solving a brainteaser or riddle doesn't cost us anything except pride or perhaps mild frustration when the answer becomes obvious (as in boxing; strawberries; dwell, dwarf, and dwindle; and Niagara Falls, the rim of which erodes roughly two-and-a-half feet each year from the millions of gallons of water that rush over it every minute).

Guesswork when it comes to raising children isn't fun, however. It carries far greater consequences and frustrations for parents and children alike. Yet for far too many parents, their parenting plan consists of hoping "this" new parenting fad works or wondering why "that" one doesn't.

What I love about Dr. Larimore's book is that he doesn't leave us with brainteasers or hope-filled guesses when it comes to the task of raising highly healthy and happy children. He gives clear, wise, accurate advice on ten tangible, everyday actions and attitudes every parent can put into practice to make a difference in a child's life.

Dr. Larimore takes the guesswork out of being a parent by blending insightful scholarship with practical applications any parent can follow. While case studies and current research abound, you'll find shoe-leather applications on protecting your child's health, nurturing close-knit relationships, keeping a parenting journal, and raising caring, confident children who can connect well with others.

There are two other things my wife and I found to be particularly helpful in Dr. Larimore's work. First, this is a guilt-free zone when it comes to understanding what makes happy, healthy children. We parents are not browbeaten with scare tactics or shamed for what we haven't done but are wisely and positively shown where to start today to become better parents. And with all his medical training and hands-on work with thousands of parents and children, Dr. Larimore knows that health for a child requires a real, growing spiritual life as well. He unashamedly urges parents to nurture a love for God into the fabric of their home and has done so with his own children.

So if you're a parent—or have a loved one or close friend who is—get this book. It will not only take the frustrating guesswork out of positive parenting, but in Doc's words, it will help you raise "highly healthy" kids in every way.

John Trent, Ph.D.,
president, StrongFamilies.com

Acknowledgments

I am grateful to the many people who have contributed to this book. The staff at Zondervan, as always, has been both professional and encouraging. Cindy Lambert has been the shepherd for each book I've written. She has been a confidante, cheerleader, and critic. Her caring, coaching, and camaraderie have provided a valued gift. Her hand-holding and encouragement during every phase of this book's development were critical. Cindy is more than a superb editor; she has become a special friend.

Dirk Buursma, as usual, has pulled the final manuscript together beautifully. As a reader of this book, you will be the recipient of his commitment to high-quality editing. Sue Brower and her staff provide the marketing and public relations services that allow this book to get into the hands of as many parents as possible.

During my four years of practice in Bryson City, North Carolina, and my sixteen years in Kissimmee, Florida, my medical partners never ceased to teach me what it meant to be a physician who inculcates highly healthy habits into the children and parents for whom he cares. Rick Pyeritz, M.D., and John Hartman, M.D., were marvelous teachers, splendid partners, trusted confidants, and brilliant physicians. They were the family physicians for my children as they grew up, and I will forever appreciate their love and care for Kate and Scott. They are two of my dearest friends, and much of this book was cultivated while I was in practice with them.

During my years of medical practice, I was privileged to deliver more than 1,500 children. I was honored to care for them and thousands of others as they grew and developed. Some are now in college and graduate school; others have married and are beginning their families. The experience I gained, at their expense and with their teaching, benefits you because I learned many of these principles from them. I'm so thankful to each of them. Whenever I share their stories here, I've taken care to protect their privacy.

Stephen and Amanda Sorenson are more than collaborating authors for this work. They have become special friends. They have labored far more on this manuscript than they ever imagined they would. I handed them a mountain of medical evidence and stories, and out of that they have crafted a document any parent can use to raise a highly healthy child.

My executive assistant, Donna Lewis, unselfishly assisted in manuscript review and research arrangements. Thanks, Donna, for your customary "above and beyond" work and dedication. Rob Flanegin and Chris Baur envisioned and built the website (www.highlyhealthy.net), which Dr. Brad Beck, Barb Seibert, Char Carter, and Charlene Vernon helped me maintain. Diane Passno and Ken Janzen at Focus on the Family spent hours reviewing the manuscript and making valuable suggestions.

Paul Batura provided extensive research to find and document portions of the medical research that I frequently used but could not cite. George Barna graciously allowed me to use his spiritual assessment tool. Bobbie Pingaro kindly permitted me to use her poem *The Meanest Mother.*

I am indebted to the Christian Medical Association for their initiative in bringing the "Highly Healthy" books to print. David Stevens, M.D., and Gene Rudd, M.D., through their leadership roles, were actively involved in bringing this project to fruition. Many thanks to those who took time to carefully review early drafts of the manuscript and offer suggestions that have improved the final product: Bruce Bagley, M.D., Patti Brown, Byron Calhoun, M.D., Reg Finger, M.D., Patti Francis, M.D., Jeff Ginther, M.D., Libby Ginther, Bernard Grunstra, M.D., Ned Hallowell, M.D., Julian Hsu, M.D., Kendra Lindberg, Tom Nevin, Peter Nieman, M.D., Phil Swihart, Chris Twiggs, and Paul Williams, M.D.

I have great appreciation for the staff at Kanakuk Kamps Colorado, who allowed me to stay at their beautiful facility near Durango to complete this book. Andy and Jamie Jo Braner were gracious hosts. Office staff members Allison King and Emily Hicks offered invaluable administrative assistance to me during my week in the Colorado Rockies.

My deepest professional acknowledgment is due my good friend David Larson, M.D. Before his untimely death in 2001, David founded and led the National Institute of Healthcare Research. We met during my residency at Duke during the late 1970s and then lost contact until the early 1990s, when David became a mentor for my research, speaking, and writing on the topic of spiritual care in clinical medicine. He was generous with his time and teaching. His friendship was a priceless gift.

I owe a special acknowledgment to Dr. James Dobson. As a young parent and husband I depended on Dr. Dobson's practical advice on parenting via his books and video series. The first time I met Jim in the fall of 1994, I told him, "If my kids are messed up, it's your fault!" He and I both laughed. For the last three years it has been my joy to be his colleague at Focus on the Family. Much of the advice and many of the stories in this book originated in the wisdom he first gave to Barb and me.

I'm thankful for Bill and Jane Judge, the experienced mentors on whom Barb and I depended as we raised our children. The two of them, who had raised five highly healthy children, would counsel us and answer our questions. They helped us become a healthier family.

I want to acknowledge the love, prayers, support, and encouragement of my best friend of more than forty-seven years and my wife of thirty years, Barb. All she's done and sacrificed to make it possible for me to write cannot be overstated. Barb, I love you.

To Kate and Scott, the two children God gave to Barb and me, I owe my gratitude for allowing me to share their stories. In many ways they were my most accomplished professors in what it means to nurture highly healthy children. Now I am the grateful father of two very highly healthy young adults. Being their father is one of the most wonderful privileges of my life.

Finally, I am grateful to God for allowing me to serve him through writing. My deepest prayer is that this work will bring glory to him and his health principles to you.

Walt Larimore, M.D.
Colorado Springs, Colorado,
June 2003

Introduction

I've written this book for moms and dads who want to raise highly healthy children. To help you do this, I'll share the advice, stories, and experiences of physicians I admire and patients I've cared for and respected. I'll share pertinent medical research and unashamedly highlight time-tested, health-related principles from the Bible. Together, we'll explore not only what makes children highly healthy but also what practical things you can do to maintain, encourage, and protect your children's growth, development, and health.

I've come to believe that, in order to raise highly healthy children, we must pay attention to ten essential principles. At first you may question whether several of these essentials deeply affect children's health, but you'll soon discover why they do.

1. Be Proactive in Preventing Physical Disease
2. Build Your Child's Health Care Team
3. Ensure Proper Nutrition
4. Provide Adequate Protection
5. Nurture Family Relationships
6. Establish a Spiritual Foundation
7. Connect with the Larger Community
8. Instill a Balanced Self-Concept
9. Engage in Healthy Activities
10. Cultivate Growth and Maturity

Even though we'll explore each of these in depth, I want you to realize this is not a how-to manual or a ten-step guidebook. Rather, these essentials are designed for and should be programmed into the very core of every parent who desires to be a great parent. If you understand these essentials and learn how to incorporate them into your family lifestyle, you will be much better prepared to raise highly healthy children. But please remember that raising a highly healthy child takes more than knowledge; it requires action—your action! Putting into practice the essential principles explained in this book is—well—essential.

GETTING THE MOST OUT OF THIS BOOK

There are at least three ways to maximize the benefits of this book. The first option is to use this simple three-step approach if you need an immediate fix:

❖ Assess your child's health.
❖ Fix the spoke that's broke.
❖ Benefit from immediate action.

Simply complete the wheel assessment in chapter 1, which will help you find the spoke that's broke. Then, using the chart on page 28, read the section that's designed to help you fix the spoke that's broke. Finally, take the recommended action.

A second option is to read through the book to get an overview and then go back to the area of greatest need and drill down. A third option is to purchase a journal or notebook and carefully read and study the book, doing the assessments and considering applications as you go. No matter which option you choose, be prepared to spend time meditating, studying, learning, and praying.

USING A JOURNAL

Using a journal as you study this book can make the difference between good intentions and actually achieving the results you desire. By journaling you'll prioritize what you want to accomplish and make your goals as specific as possible.

Purchase a journal with blank pages. On the first page, write your name and the date you begin your journey toward nurturing your highly healthy teen. Keep the journal with your book, writing notes to yourself as you read. This journal is private—for your (and your spouse's) eyes only.

As you journal, note each principle and the action you're applying, as well as each goal you're setting. Give yourself plenty of time to accomplish each goal. Making progress toward your goals—even if it's steady and slow—is more important than setting goals you can't reach.

USING THE INTERNET RECOMMENDATIONS

At times I recommend information or resources that can be accessed easily via the Internet, but I haven't provided the Internet addresses for two reasons: (1) Web addresses tend to change over time, and (2) I may find better sites in the future. Therefore, I built an Internet site (www.highlyhealthy.net) you'll be able to visit at no cost. At www.highlyhealthy.net, you'll find a list of each of the sites I've recommended. By double-clicking on these listings, you'll be taken to the most up-to-date site for the information or health tools you need.

This site will be updated as often as needed and will host not only *God's Design for the Highly Healthy Child* but also *God's Design for the Highly Healthy Person* and *God's Design for the Highly Healthy Teen*, as well as any other *Highly Healthy* tools, books, or newsletters that may be developed in the future.

PART ONE

The

FOUNDATION
FOR HEALTH

Chapter One

What Is a Highly Healthy Child?

Eight-year-old Daryl was an impressive young boy. I don't think I've ever met a person with a more positive mind-set. His attitude was always upbeat, his laugh infectious. I wish you could have seen his smile. It could light up even the darkest room. Daryl was loved by his family and had a deep faith in God. In short, he was incredibly healthy emotionally, relationally, and spiritually. He was more highly healthy than most of my patients, and more healthy than most people I had met.

Daryl's overall health was all the more impressive because of where I met him. He was visiting "Give Kids the World," a special village near Disney World where dying children and their families can escape the world of hospitals and medical treatments and enjoy a week of being lavished with hugs, smiles, and entertainment from their favorite Disney characters. Although Daryl was as bald as a cucumber and skin and bones from end-stage cancer, he was living life to the fullest. He greatly expanded my understanding of health. He demonstrated what it means to be healthy—not just disease and symptom free, but *whole* in the most important ways.

WHAT IS HEALTH?

Because I was trained in conventional medicine, I initially emphasized the physical side of health, especially the treatment of trauma and disease. If my patients were free from injury and disease, I considered them to be healthy.

But the longer I practiced medicine and the more I encountered individuals like Daryl, the more I realized there's more to being highly healthy than having a physically functioning body. All the evidence suggests that true health involves our entire beings, with all elements—physical, emotional, relational, and spiritual—functioning as God designed them to function if we are to be truly healthy.

Dose of Wisdom

When the physical, mental, and spiritual dimensions of well-being are singing in harmony, you're healthy. That doesn't mean there is no room for a dissonant chord, but that the music of life is pleasant to the ear.

Nick Zervanos, M.D., family physician

The well-being of highly healthy children depends on their inner life as well as their physical health. God wants to nourish and promote a healthy emotional, relational, and spiritual life because without it, our children simply will be less healthy than God designed them to be (Proverbs 17:22; Matthew 5:3–12; 6:33; 16:26; Luke 6:20–26; and 1 Corinthians 11:29–30 are just a few Bible passages that support this statement).

Let's turn now to explore what I call the "four wheels of health" and discover why each is so important in helping children achieve the highest possible degree of health.

UNDERSTANDING THE FOUR WHEELS OF HEALTH

In order to understand how to nurture our children's health, we need to understand a concept taught to me by Harold, who lived in a small cabin on a hill above the Nantahala River near Bryson City, North Carolina. Harold's true joy in life was refurbishing Model T Fords. To him, they were works of art. When I expressed an interest in learning more about these old cars, Harold invited me to his shop, where I gained a greater appreciation for his hobby.

Harold labored over body repairs and reupholstering seats, but he specialized in repairing wheels. He showed me how a weakness in just one or two spokes could cause a multispoked wheel to collapse and, potentially, cause a wreck. He explained that if a driver wanted a long, smooth ride, the wheels needed to be as perfectly balanced as possible. An imbalance in even one wheel could put a strain on the engine, chassis, and other wheels. In short, it could goof up the whole car.

I began to think about the components of health in the way Harold viewed the components of a sturdy wheel: four wheels attached to a stable car (the four health "wheels" of a highly healthy person), with all wheels in balance (all aspects of a highly healthy child developed in balance). The four "wheels" of highly healthy children are

- **physical health**—the well-being of a child's body;
- **emotional health**—the well-being of a child's mental faculties and connection with his or her emotions;
- **relational health**—the well-being of a child's associations with parents, family members, friends, and community; and
- **spiritual health**—the well-being of a child's relationship with God

These four components of health were critical in the life of Jesus, even during childhood. According to the Bible, Jesus "grew in wisdom and stature, and in favor with God and men." In other words, he grew mentally/emotionally, physically, spiritually, and relationally.

Parents who want to raise highly healthy children will work hard to keep the wheels of their health and those of their children in balance. So let's consider the effect of each of the four wheels of health and explore the essential principles you can begin implementing to raise a highly healthy child.

The Physical Wheel

The simplest definition of maximum physical health is that the child's body—all its chemicals, parts, and systems—is working as closely as possible to the way God designed it. In order for a child to be physically healthy, disease must be prevented whenever possible and treated as early as possible. When illness or disorder occurs, physical health involves learning to cope and adapt as needed. With good emotional, relational, and spiritual health, a child whose body lacks optimum physical "wholeness" can still be highly healthy.

Allow me to share a personal illustration. Our oldest child, Kate, was born with cerebral palsy. Most of her right brain and about one-half of her left brain died and dissolved while she was in the womb. Kate's brain damage was such that it was as though she had had a stroke before she was born—resulting in the left side of her body being weaker and more spastic than the right side (although the right side, too, was affected). The brain damage dramatically slowed her physical development. By the time she was a teenager, she had had many operations to straighten her limbs and eyes. She had worn braces and splints, casts and eye patches, and for a time she was in a wheelchair. At the age of twelve, she developed a severe seizure disorder. She spent time in an intensive care unit on a ventilator and nearly died.

Although Kate made it through many medical obstacles, she is still not "normal" physically. She has significant disabilities, and her condition is incurable. Nevertheless, she has learned to cope and adapt. Although she doesn't eat as well as she might and could exercise a bit more, for the most part she cares for herself physically. Kate is up-to-date on her immunizations. She takes her medications, makes her doctor appointments, and does her own self-care. Her mom and I consider her physical wheel to be fairly healthy—not because her health is perfect but because it is reasonably balanced.

Given her physical challenges, it would be easy for Kate to become unhealthy. I've known patients with similar disabilities who were very unhealthy emotionally, relationally, or spiritually. They were miserable people. They became obese, and their physical health was terrible. So Kate's physical health cannot be taken for granted. It takes a concerted effort on her part to maintain her physical wheel, and her physical health is strongly dependent on the constant work she does to keep her emotional, relational, and spiritual wheels in balance. If these three wheels were flattened, weak, or unbalanced, Kate couldn't be nearly as healthy as she is physically.

The Emotional Wheel

Great emotional health is not the absence of emotional distress. Emotional health involves learning to cope with and then embrace the full spectrum of human emotions—positive and negative—we all face in life. Emotional health in children is greatly enhanced by the love, security, and well-defined boundaries of the parent-child relationship. On the foundation of our love, we parents must teach our children how to appropriately recognize and express the full range of human emotions. Four-year-old Samuel, the child of a friend, surprised me with the level of emotional health he demonstrated one day in our home.

Samuel's little sister crawled over to where he was playing with a train set. She sat up and reached over to take one of the cars.

"Rachel, I wish you wouldn't do that." He glared at her.

She looked him in the face, then grabbed one of the train cars and pulled it into her lap.

We watched to see what Samuel would do.

He fumed for a moment. "Rachel," he continued, "if you put the train back on the track, we can play together."

I was quite amazed by this little boy's maturity.

Then Rachel surprised us all. She took the little train car and banged it on her brother's head!

He grimaced. Had he been my child, I would have bolted to his side to attempt to prevent the coming eruption. Samuel's mom, however, sat and watched.

He looked up with tears forming in his eyes. Then he stood and walked to his mom. "Mommy, Rachel hit me on the head."

"How did that make you feel?" she asked.

"I felt really, really, really angry, and my insides wanted to punch her."

"Why didn't you?"

"I knew it was wrong."

She hugged him tightly. "Samuel I love you so much—no matter what decisions you make. But I'm so very proud of this decision. You and I will do something special together as soon as we get home."

At his young age, Samuel was well on his way to being emotionally healthy. His response was not natural behavior; it was learned. His parents had taught him principles on which he now acted. He was fully aware of his feelings and made a conscious decision as to how he would respond.

The Relational Wheel

Great relational or social health can be defined as the state of maximum well-being in all of a child's relationships—those with siblings, parents, relatives, friends, schoolmates, teachers, coaches, clergy, neighbors, and the broader community. Early on, relational health requires parents to involve their children in healthy relationships and protect them from toxic or dangerous relationships. As children mature, it involves teaching them how to exercise discernment in their relationships.

Although relational stress and discord are inevitable as children learn to interact with other people, it's critical to our children's well-being that we parents learn how to develop healthy relationships ourselves and that we be diligent in preventing or "treating" disordered relationships to which our children will be exposed (including our own). Our relationships do have a direct impact on our children for better or for worse. Marshall stands out as an example of how parental relationships affect the relational health of a child.

When my wife, Barb, and I lived in Bryson City, we taught the young boys' Sunday school class. One of the boys, Marshall, was a gifted athlete. He was full of spunk and energy. He was intellectually gifted and seemed to grasp spiritual truth. But he was a deeply wounded child. No one in Marshall's family had learned how to have healthy relationships, so the entire family was involved in toxic relationships. His father was an alcoholic who, we believe, abused Marshall in terrible ways. His oldest brother was a delinquent. His mom was physically weak and lived in constant pain—a pain she took out on her kids.

These extremely disordered relationships affected Marshall emotionally and flowed over into his relationships with others. It wasn't surprising that by the time we met Marshall, his interactions with other children were characterized by either anger or selfishness. While other children accepted correction, Marshall rebelled. While other children followed instructions, Marshall disobeyed. It was no wonder he was failing in school.

As concerned adults, Barb and I poured much time into Marshall. We tried to help him balance this unhealthy wheel. We knew that if we couldn't help him develop a strategy for balancing it, the road ahead most likely would be rough. And indeed it was. He eventually dropped out of school and became an alcoholic.

The Spiritual Wheel

Although not everyone shares my view, I'm convinced the spiritual wheel is the most crucial. Good physical, emotional, and relational health aren't enough. Spiritual well-being needs to be nurtured from an early age so it'll be a consistent priority of children who will become highly healthy adults.

Great spiritual health can be described as the state of a child's maximum well-being in a personal relationship with God the Creator. To be spiritually healthy, a child needs to be taught what a personal relationship with God is and to see other people model that kind of relationship. Then the child must choose to have this type of relationship with God. Finally, he or she must grow in this relationship over time—just as in any other relationship.

Even very young children need to learn about God's plan for them in terms of their physical, emotional, relational, and spiritual conditions. They must learn about their Creator's personal instruction and direction in their lives, and they must learn how to apply it in simple, practical ways.

One mother told me about taking a walk with her two-year-old daughter. They sat down for a rest, and the child looked up at the sky and said, "'Ky. God make 'ky."

"Yes, God made the sky," her mother replied.

The wind gently rustled nearby tree branches. The child said, "Trees. God make trees."

"Yes, God made the trees," her mother replied.

Just then a bird flew by. "Birdie. Grammie Rosie make birdies!"

"Oh!" her mother laughed. "Grammie Rosie makes lots of things for you that are soft and fluffy like birdies, but God makes the birdies, just like he makes the trees and sky."

Making the nurturing of spiritual health a priority in everyday life is essential, especially because so many people view physical, emotional, relational, and even financial health as their top priorities. Children often receive this message from schoolmates, advertisements, movies, and their interactions with adults, but it's *not* a view held by parents of highly healthy children. These parents echo Jesus' perspective when he said the most important thing is to seek God's kingdom and his righteousness, and that the material needs of food and clothing would then follow. These parents ask, as did Jesus, "What good will it be for a man [child] if he gains the whole world, yet forfeits his soul?"

Does my emphasis on spiritual health mean that physical, emotional, and relational health aren't important? Certainly not! All these aspects should be enjoyed and appreciated, nurtured and developed. Nevertheless, if the spiritual wheel receives less attention than the other three wheels, our children will not be highly healthy. Nor will they grow up to be highly healthy adults unless they develop this wheel on their own. Balance in all four health wheels is essential. Sadly, many people put the spare tire on the car and toss the spiritual wheel in the trunk!

Dose of Wisdom

Man must be arched and buttressed from within; else the temple wavers to the dust.

Roman Emperor Marcus Aurelius

ASSESSING YOUR CHILD'S HEALTH

I believe you want to help your child become as highly healthy as possible, so I'll share an easy way to assess the four wheels of health for each of your children. I designed this measurement tool for children approximately ages four to twelve. It's simple—and as such it will be only a crude representation of your child's overall health—but it will help you quickly develop a picture of your child's health balance, or lack thereof. Understanding these wheels is fairly simple, and using them to evaluate your child is fairly intuitive. So let's begin. On a separate sheet of paper, reproduce or copy this simple illustration:

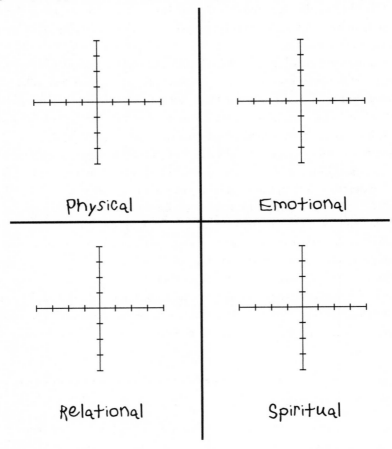

Notice that each of the four health wheels has a hub and two sets of spokes. The hub is the central point around which the entire wheel turns, and it involves faith—not in the religious sense but in terms of the confidence that if you provide what your child needs to be healthy, he or she will most likely become healthier over time. The spokes represent the measure of health your child possesses in each of these areas. The longer the spoke, the better. In this exercise, you'll assess the length of each spoke of each wheel, which will show how smooth a ride your child will enjoy on the road to health.

Warning! *Don't* use this exercise to show your child where he or she comes up short. To do so could be highly damaging to your child. This tool is designed for your eyes only—to show where *you* need to improve in order to raise a healthier child. This measurement tool hasn't been scientifically verified. My guidance on measuring these spokes is based on both my experience and my review of the research literature.

As you read each description, mark the appropriate spoke to represent your evaluation of your child's health in this area. The more accurately you assess your child, the more helpful this tool will be. The hub is the zero point.

Physical Wheel

Hub = trust that your child's body will develop properly if nurtured
Vertical Spokes = activity and rest
Horizontal Spokes = nutrition/growth and immunizations

Activity

This spoke, the top one on the wheel, represents your child's average physical activity over the last two or three months.

- Full spoke: My child exercises (runs, walks, plays outside, or participates in sports or physical education) at least thirty minutes six or seven days a week.
- 3/4 spoke: My child exercises at least thirty minutes per day, four or five days a week.
- 1/2 spoke: My child exercises at least thirty minutes per day, three days a week.
- 1/4 spoke: My child exercises only one or two days a week or less than thirty minutes a day.
- No spoke: My child is a couch potato. He or she participates in no physical education at school and no sports activities.

Rest

On average, over the last two to three months, how would you assess your child's sleep and rest habits? Consider these factors for the bottom spoke:

1. My child goes to bed at a reasonable hour.

2. My child gets eight or more hours of restful sleep most nights of the week.
3. My child usually wakes up refreshed.
4. My child has time every day for play, rest, and recreation.
5. My child enjoys one or more adequate, restful family vacations each year.

- Full spoke: My child achieves five of the above.
- 3/4 spoke: My child achieves four of the above.
- 1/2 spoke: My child achieves three of the above.
- 1/4 spoke: My child achieves two of the above.
- No spoke: My child achieves zero or one of the above.

Now let's turn our attention from the vertical spokes of the physical health wheel to its horizontal spokes.

Nutrition/Growth

The left-hand spoke represents your child's nutritional health and growth. Each component accounts for no more than one-half of the spoke.

First, let's assess the *nutrition* portion of the spoke. Consider these factors:

1. My child drinks plenty of water daily.
2. My child eats at least two to four servings of fruits and three to five servings of vegetables daily.
3. My child eats at least three nutritious meals per day.
4. My child has minimal intake of caffeine and soft drinks.
5. My child has minimal intake of saturated fats and highly processed foods.
6. My child has fewer than two or three fast-food meals a month.
7. My child is rarely exposed to secondhand smoke.

- 1/2 spoke: My child does six or seven of the above.
- 1/4 spoke: My child does four or five of the above.
- No spoke: My child does less than four of the above.

Now let's consider your child's *growth*. If your child is two years old or older, the most accurate assessment of healthy growth is the Body Mass Index (BMI). Ask your child's doctor for a BMI chart for children or use the chart on my website (www.highlyhealthy.net).

- 1/2 spoke: My child's BMI is normal.
- 1/4 spoke: My child's BMI is borderline.
- No spoke: My child's BMI is abnormally high or low.

Your final mark on this spoke should be the sum of the nutrition and growth marks.

Immunizations

Of all the preventive measures available to positively influence our children's physical health, this one may be the most essential. I'll discuss the importance of immunizations in chapter 3. To measure this spoke, determine how many recommended immunizations your child has received. You can find a list on my website (www.highlyhealthy.net).

- Full spoke: My child has received all recommended vaccines.
- 3/4 spoke: My child has received between 75 and 100 percent of the recommended vaccines.
- 1/2 spoke: My child has received between 50 and 75 percent of the recommended vaccines.
- 1/4 spoke: My child has received between 25 and 50 percent of the recommended vaccines.
- No spoke: My child has received less than 25 percent of the recommended vaccines.

Emotional Wheel

Hub = trust that your child's emotions will develop properly if nurtured
Vertical spokes = love/respect and affirmation/appreciation
Horizontal spokes = media/learning and boundaries

Love/Respect

Consider these factors for the top spoke of this wheel:

1. I frequently communicate to my child that I love him or her.
2. I enjoy reading and talking to my child in a warm and friendly voice.
3. I try to show interest and enthusiasm when my child is speaking. I pay attention when he or she talks to me—even if it means stopping what I'm doing.

4. I feel emotionally warm and affectionate toward my child and hug or hold him or her frequently.

5. I consciously look for things to admire, respect, and appreciate about my child.

6. I look for opportunities to find my child doing things correctly and well.

A. I feel my love for my child is most frequently unconditional—that my love is not withheld based on behavior, performance, or looks. (Of course, it doesn't mean you always like the behavior, but it does mean you always love your child "in spite of ...," even when you detest the behavior.)

B. I feel my love for my child is most frequently conditional—that my love is predicated on how my child behaves, performs, or looks (love "if ..." or "because of ...").

- Full spoke: I believe all six of the numbered factors above are true.
- 3/4 spoke: I believe five of the numbered factors above are true.
- 1/2 spoke: I believe four of the numbered factors above are true.
- 1/4 spoke: I believe two or three of the numbered factors above are true.
- No spoke: I believe zero or one of the numbered factors above apply to me and my child.
- Add up to 1/2 spoke if A is true.
- Subtract up to 1/2 spoke if B is true.

Why do I give so much credence to the type of love we choose to give our child? As we'll explore in chapter 10, a key foundation for a highly healthy child is unconditional love, which helps reduce a child's risk for immature anger, resentment, guilt, depression, anxiety, insecurity, and many other highly unhealthy factors. Unconditional love balances love with discipline, freedom with limits, and nurture with training. Such a relationship will be healthy, enjoyable, and affectionate for both of you—which leads to the other vertical spoke.

Affirmation/Appreciation

Consider the following factors for the bottom spoke:

1. I am my child's best cheerleader. I frequently praise my child and tell my child I appreciate what he or she has done and that I believe in him or her.

2. I hug my child frequently and often tell my child how much I appreciate him or her.

3. I thank my child for doing things without my asking, and I demonstrate my gratitude for the little things he or she does.

4. I desire to spend time with my child and enjoy being with him or her.

5. My child is comfortable coming to me when he or she is experiencing joy, satisfaction, guilt, shame, sadness, or a host of other emotions.

6. My child frequently talks with me and enjoys being with me. I try to listen to my child without preaching, judging, or criticizing. I listen to my child with the intent to just listen.

7. I understand my child's temperament, talents, and love language. I let my child know about the unique qualities, gifts, and talents I admire in him or her.

8. I know what my child is capable of achieving, and I help my child set goals based on what is appropriate for him or her as a unique individual.

- Full spoke: I believe eight of the above are true.
- 3/4 spoke: I believe six or seven of the above are true.
- 1/2 spoke: I believe four or five of the above are true.
- 1/4 spoke: I believe two or three of the above are true.
- No spoke: I believe zero or one of the above apply to me and my child.

Researchers call these two vertical spokes the "parental warmth" or "parental receptiveness" spokes. They deal with your expression of verbal and physical affection toward your child, as well as your praise and acceptance.

Now we'll turn from the vertical spokes of the emotional health wheel to its horizontal spokes.

Media/Learning

To come up with the measurement for this left-hand spoke, add the following two factors together.

The first half of the left-hand spoke is your child's exposure to media. One could make the argument that today's children are overstimulated. More often than not, too much media in children's lives—video games, computer games, and way too much television—assaults their senses, negatively affects their minds, and is detrimental to their emotions and body. Many media providers are trying to influence our children in ways that most parents consider highly unhealthy. Highly healthy parents know how to set limits when it comes to media. Where does your child line up?

- 1/2 spoke: Our home is TV free or my child watches one hour or less a day, and the computer/Internet is only used in a public area of our home and for educational purposes. If my child watches TV, I routinely monitor what he or she watches. I monitor what my child does on the Internet.
- 1/4 spoke: My child is routinely exposed to two hours or less a day of media (television, videos, video games, and computer activities). Also, I sometimes monitor what my child watches on TV and does on the Internet.
- No spoke: My child is routinely exposed to two to four or more hours a day of media, or I never monitor what my child watches on TV and does on the Internet.
- Subtract up to 1/4 spoke if your child has a TV in his or her bedroom or unfettered Internet access in the bedroom.

The second half of this left-hand spoke is your child's enjoyment of learning and mental activity. Research shows that the brain, like a muscle, must be exercised in order to remain highly healthy. Just as physical activity helps a child's physiological structure stay healthy, stimulating mental activity benefits his or her brain. Activities such as reading, doing crossword puzzles, and even playing board games with family members have been linked with sharper minds throughout life. So how much does your child like to learn?

- 1/2 spoke: My child shows a moderate to high level of enjoyment for mental activities such as reading, ongoing education and learning, challenging mental tasks, good conversation, or board games with the family.
- 1/4 spoke: My child shows little enjoyment for mental activities and learning.
- No spoke: My child shows almost no enjoyment for mental activities and learning.

Boundaries

Reducing the media your child is exposed to and setting appropriate expectations and limits compose what researchers call "parental demandingness." When balanced with parental warmth (the love spokes), a child is more likely to be highly healthy. Too much of one or too little of the other leads to reduced levels of health.

"Parental demandingness" (discipline, expectations, and coaching) is the extent to which a child's parents expect responsible behavior from their child and maintain what the researchers call a "hands-on attitude." This includes consistently setting and enforcing rules or limits on your child. Rules for children, however, must be clear, reasonable, developmentally appropriate, fair and just, mutually agreed upon, and flexible—emphasizing what to do rather than just what not to do.

Measure this spoke based on how many of the following boundaries you consistently impose:

1. I routinely know where my child is after school and on weekends.
2. I expect to be and am told the truth by my child about where he or she is really going.
3. I am aware of my child's academic performance and visit with his or her teachers from time to time.
4. I eat dinner with my child at least five times a week.
5. I eat breakfast with my child at least five times a week.
6. I assign my child regular chores.
7. I turn off the TV during dinner and rarely eat in front of the TV.
8. There is an adult present whenever my child returns from school.

- Full spoke: I believe all eight of the above are true.
- 3/4 spoke: I believe six or seven of the above are true.
- 1/2 spoke: I believe four or five of the above are true.
- 1/4 spoke: I believe two or three of the above are true.
- No spoke: I believe zero or one of the above applies to me and my child.

Relational Wheel

Hub = trust in and nurturing healthy relationships with others and self
Vertical Spokes = relationship with parents and family relationships
Horizontal Spokes = connectedness and performance in school/
                extracurricular activities

Relationship with Parents

Of all the characteristics of highly healthy parents, other than loving your children unconditionally, the most important is the quantity of time you sacrificially give to your child. Your relationship with your child is critical to his or her self-concept and ability to develop and maintain healthy relationships. A crucial measure of your relationship is the amount of time you spend with your child. Use these factors to mark the top spoke of this wheel:

- Full spoke: Both my spouse and I spend more than thirty minutes each day with our child(ren).
- 3/4 spoke: Either my spouse or I spend more than thirty minutes each day with our child(ren); the other spends between two and three hours each week with our child(ren).
- 1/2 spoke: Both my spouse and I spend between two and three hours each week with our child(ren).
- 1/4 spoke: Both my spouse and I spend some time but less than two hours weekly with our child(ren).
- No spoke: Neither my spouse nor I spend any significant time with our child(ren).

Family Relationships

The relationship between a child's parents, as I'll show later, is a critical factor in the life of a highly healthy child. What is the quality of family relationships around your child? Use these factors to mark the bottom spoke of this wheel:

For married, biological parents who live together

- Full spoke: My spouse and I have a great marriage.
- 3/4 spoke: My spouse and I have a moderately good marriage.
- 1/2 spoke: My spouse and I have a marriage fair in quality.
- 1/4 spoke: My spouse and I have a marriage of poor quality.

For married parents of adopted children who live together

- 3/4 spoke: My spouse and I have a great marriage.
- 1/2 spoke: My spouse and I have a moderately good marriage.
- 1/4 spoke: My spouse and I have a marriage fair in quality
- No spoke: My spouse and I have a marriage of poor quality.

For single parents

- Full spoke: I spend more than thirty minutes each day with my child. I also involve positive, significant role models of the opposite gender (of the single parent) in my child's life three hours or more each week.

- 3/4 spoke: I spend more than thirty minutes each day with my child. I also involve positive, significant role models of the opposite gender (of the single parent) in my child's life at least one hour each week.
- 1/2 spoke: I spend at least thirty minutes each day with my child. I have not yet provided positive, significant role models of the opposite gender (of the single parent) for my child.
- 1/4 spoke: I spend less than thirty minutes each day with my child. I have not yet provided positive, significant role models of the opposite gender (of the single parent) for my child.
- No spoke: I spend less than two hours each week with my child. I have not yet provided positive, significant role models of the opposite gender (of the single parent) for my child.

For parents in blended families

- Full spoke: My relationship with my spouse and my stepchildren is great, and we have five or more years under our belts.
- 3/4 spoke: My relationship with my spouse and my stepchildren is great, and we have less than five years under our belts.
- 1/2 spoke: My relationship with my spouse and my stepchildren is only moderately good.
- 1/4 spoke: My relationship with my spouse and my stepchildren is fair to poor.
- No spoke: My child and I are in a blended family, but I am not married.

Now we'll take into account the horizontal spokes of the relational wheel.

Connectedness

A child's connectedness to his or her parents and friends is foundational to his or her relational as well as emotional health (since relational and emotional health are intricately interwoven). Connectedness in the parent-child relationship begins with affirmation, blameless (unconditional) love, and boundaries, which we've already measured as part of the emotional wheel. Children with healthy levels of connectedness not only have strong relationships with good friends or playmates; they also exhibit a willingness to interact constructively with others, a can-do attitude, a willingness to tackle new adventures, a sense of optimism, and an ability to make friends comfortably.

Add the following two factors to measure the left-hand spoke:

Connectedness with friends or playmates

- 1/2 spoke: My child has terrific relationships and plays well with others.
- 1/4 spoke: My child has fair to moderately good relationships with his or her friends or sometimes doesn't play well with others.
- No spoke: My child either has poor, negative relationships with his or her friends, or my child usually doesn't play well with others.

Attitudes

1. My child displays a can-do attitude.
2. My child displays a willingness to tackle new adventures.
3. My child displays a sense of optimism.
4. My child displays an ability to make friends comfortably.

- 1/2 spoke: My child displays four of the above factors.
- 1/4 spoke: My child displays two or three of the above factors.
- No spoke: My child displays zero or one of the above factors.

Performance in School/Extracurricular Activities

Rate this spoke by the meaningfulness of your child's "work"—how he or she is doing in school. Given individual talents, how much is he or she achieving? How is your child doing in extracurricular activities? Does your child participate in at least one healthy activity—a club, sport, or church activity—that gives him or her satisfaction? For this spoke add the "Performance in School" and "Extracurricular Activities" scores together.

Performance in school

Given my child's gifts, temperament, and talents—

- 1/2 spoke: My child is performing as competently as he or she can.
- 1/4 spoke: My child is performing with some competence but not as competently as he or she can.
- No spoke: My child isn't performing nearly as competently as he or she can.

Extracurricular activities

- 1/2 spoke: My child participates in at least two healthy activities—club, sport, or church activity—that gives him or her satisfaction.
- 1/4 spoke: My child has one healthy activity—a club, sport, or church activity—that gives him or her satisfaction.
- No spoke: My child is not involved in healthy extracurricular activities.

Spiritual Wheel

Hub = trust in and nurturing a healthy relationship with God
Vertical Spokes = personal relationship with God and prayer
Horizontal Spokes = spiritual instruction and spiritual activity

Personal Relationship with God

I define true, positive spirituality in terms of a personal relationship with God resulting in an internal change that yields love, joy, peace, patience, kindness, goodness, faithfulness, gentleness, and self-control. However, these traits can take years to develop and are not at all natural to children—even if they have a close relationship with God. As I'll discuss in chapter 8, the greater the depth of a child's spiritual health, the more likely the child is to be physically, emotionally, and relationally healthy. This can be difficult to assess, especially in young children, but it's worth it to give it your best shot.

- Full spoke: My child believes in God and shows evidence of an extremely close relationship with God.
- 3/4 spoke: My child believes in God and shows evidence of a moderately good relationship with God.
- 1/2 spoke: My child believes in God and shows evidence of some relationship with God.
- 1/4 spoke: My child believes in God but doesn't seem to have a personal relationship with God.
- No spoke: My child has no relationship with and no belief in God.

Prayer

In its simplest form, prayer is an intimate conversation between your child and his or her Creator. Prayer can occur anywhere and anytime. It doesn't require a church or synagogue, a particular place or position. Prayer can be as simple as thanking God for the good things that happen each day. How often does your child pray?

- Full spoke: My child prays every day.
- 3/4 spoke: My child prays only a few days each week.
- 1/2 spoke: My child prays only a few times each month.
- 1/4 spoke: My child prays only on special holidays or before family meals.
- No spoke: My child never prays or prays only during a crisis.

Spiritual Instruction

The foundation for spiritual health is most effectively laid during childhood and must include spiritual instruction. Activities such as family Bible reading, Sunday school classes, confirmation classes, vacation Bible school, church camp, and the like all play a role in spiritual instruction. Add the "daily or weekly" and the "annual" scores together for this spoke.

Your child's *daily or weekly* religious instruction accounts for up to half a spoke.

- 1/2 spoke: My child participates in two or more activities such as attending a faith community; joining in our family's Scripture reading; and attending Sunday school classes each week.
- 1/4 spoke: My child participates in only one activity such as attending a faith community; joining in our family's Scripture reading; and attending Sunday school classes each month.
- No spoke: My child participates in no religious instruction venues.

For the other component, evaluate *annual* religious instruction.

- 1/2 spoke: My child participates in two of the following or similar activities each year: church camp, vacation Bible school, or a church play.
- 1/4 spoke: My child participates in one of the following or similar activities each year: church camp, vacation Bible school, or a church play.
- No spoke: My child participates in no annual religious instruction.

Spiritual Activity

For up to half of this spoke, evaluate your child's daily or weekly *involvement in a faith community.*

- 1/2 spoke: My child and I are involved at least weekly in a healthy, positive spiritual community in which we receive supportive guidance and practice accountability.
- 1/4 spoke: My child and I are involved less than weekly but at least monthly in a healthy, positive spiritual community in which we receive supportive guidance and practice accountability, or we are involved in a spiritual community but it's somewhat unhealthy and offers only some supportive guidance and accountability.

- No spoke: My child and I are not involved in a spiritual community at all, or we are involved in a spiritual community but it's very unhealthy and offers no supportive guidance and accountability.

The other half of this spoke focuses on *giving* to others.

- 1/2 spoke: My child gives away time, treasure, or talent at least monthly by participating in at least one of the following or similar activities: volunteering at a soup kitchen, helping a neighbor, cleaning up along a roadside, or giving money to a church or charity.
- 1/4 spoke: My child gives away time, treasure, or talent once each year by participating in at least one of the following or similar activities: volunteering at a soup kitchen, helping a neighbor, cleaning up along a roadside, or giving money to a church or charity.
- No spoke: My child does not give away time, treasure, or talent by serving others.

The Whole Picture

Now that you've marked the estimated length of the spokes on your child's four wheels of health, complete the picture by drawing a wheel from the end of each spoke. Are your child's wheels round, or are they flat in spots? If there are any severely wobbly wheels, he or she is less than highly healthy. Could he or she make it on a set of wheels like you see below from a child I know?

Now is the time to begin lengthening the short spokes of your child's wheels of health. If you take the principles in this book to heart and apply them, you'll see different spokes lengthen as you make decisions a parent who intends to raise a highly healthy child would make.

It's fine to identify the flattest wheel or the most broken spokes. To find the flattest wheel, assign a point count to each spoke of each wheel:

- Full spoke = 4 points
- 3/4 spoke = 3 point
- 1/2 spoke = 2 points
- 1/4 spoke = 1 points
- No spoke = 0 points

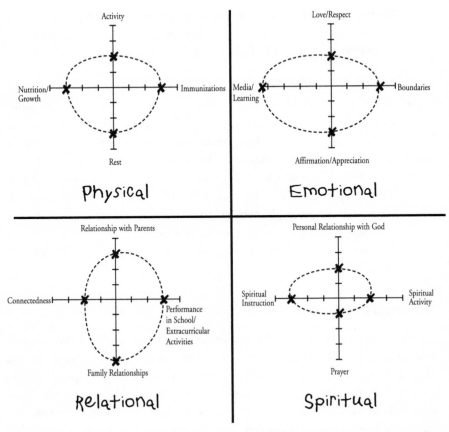

A perfectly round, fully inflated wheel will have 16 points (4 points for each spoke). In this illustration, the physical wheel has 11 points, the emotional wheel 12 points, the relational wheel 12 points, and the spiritual wheel 8 points. As you can see, this child's spiritual wheel is the least healthy

So the spiritual wheel may be the first one these parents would address. If there were equally weakened wheels, I'd urge parents to choose the wheel they think would be the easiest to fix and turn to that area of the book.

Another option is to deal with the shortest spokes. Look again at the illustration, and you'll see that the bottom spoke on the spiritual wheel is the shortest of all of this child's spokes. If your child has more than one spoke that is equally short, choose the one you consider the easiest to address and read the section in this book that deals with that wheel of health.

Whether you do something now about your child's flattened wheel(s) or short spoke(s) or read on and get an overview, this chapter can serve as a reference as you look at ways to equip your child to live a highly healthy life.

Chapter Two

The Parental Role in Nurturing a Highly Healthy Child

After completing medical school, I accepted a brief general-practice teaching fellowship at Queen's Medical Center in Nottingham, England. Following that commitment, Barb and I spent several months traveling by camping van across continental Europe and northern Africa.

One weekend, while visiting new friends in Munich, Germany, Barb became ill. Our host suggested that Barb might be pregnant. We did not think it was possible, but the next morning we scurried off to the local pharmacist and picked up one of the very early versions of the home pregnancy test. In those days, the specimen had to react for several hours before producing a readable result, so while the brew "cooked," Barb and I toured the zoo. At the appointed hour we returned to our van, opened the door, and found a very positive pregnancy test.

Shocked, Barb immediately echoed the thoughts of most prospective parents: "What do we do now?"

There's not a parent or parent-to-be who doesn't wish that pregnancy and children came with a set of instructions. I always smile when I read the Bible story about Samson's parents. Apparently his mother had been unable to have a child, but one day while she was alone in a field, an angel appeared and told her she would have a son. She hurried home to tell her husband. His response was great. He immediately prayed and asked God to send the angel back to teach them how to raise the child!

Fortunately for Samson's parents the angel did reappear. Most parents, however, don't receive the benefit of a personal consultation on child rearing with a messenger from God. Nevertheless, there are foundational principles we parents can practice to increase the likelihood that our children will not only develop normally but will become as healthy as possible. These essential principles can help us navigate the incredible responsibilities and challenges of raising children to become highly healthy adults.

THE PARENTAL TEAM

The task of raising healthy children begins with an understanding of our role as parents. We must not only learn the principles, but also have a deep desire to raise highly healthy children and then discipline ourselves to make the sacrifices necessary to do so. But please don't think you have to be a perfect parent to raise highly healthy children. No one can be a perfect parent. Barb and I certainly were not.

Nevertheless, you are absolutely essential in your child's life simply because you are your child's parent. You are the foundation on which your child builds his or her health. And parenting isn't just what we do; it is who we are committed to be. This is true not just for one parent but for both parents. Parenting is a full-time job for two. It must be "Job One" for *both* the mom and dad.

I realize I may be out of step with the times in emphasizing a "mom and dad team" approach to raising highly healthy children. After all, among industrialized nations the United States leads the world in the percentage of single parents. As of the year 2000, married families made up less than 25 percent of all households. Given these disturbing trends, it is predicted that about half of the children today will spend at least part of their childhood living in a single-parent home. Despite these trends, there are important reasons why a loving, married, two-parent (mom and dad) home is most conducive to raising highly healthy children. When such a home life is not possible, however, all is not lost. Single parents with the desire and discipline to do so can take positive steps to counteract the obstacles they face and maximize their children's health. I'll consider these steps further in chapter 7. For now, let's begin by reflecting on the ideal and discovering why it is so important to children's health.

Thousands of years of recorded human history, the wisdom of the Bible, and a huge database of medical and social science research clearly indicate that children who live in homes with their biological parents who have a stable marriage are, in general, far healthier than those who live in almost any other family arrangement or who live in a family that is about to come apart. The most highly healthy children tend to come from homes with a married mom and dad who love each other and are willing to sacrifice for the sake of the special role they have in raising children. This is the soil in which the tree of family life grows best.

A number of researchers have found that a good marriage and a close family improve the well-being of a husband and wife and seem to inoculate children against despair and many other poor mental and physical health outcomes. For example, sociologist Glen Elder found that boys and girls born during the 1920s were happier during the Great Depression if their parents had a strong marriage. Teens who grew up in strong families during hard times remained, in general, very happy as adults. Elder concluded that the strong parental relationships were "a source of resilience for kids." More recent research confirms that a good marriage helps protect children's mental health during economic hardship. These findings were even more impressive in families where "multi-generational closeness" prevailed.

A good marriage is also a significant factor in preventing drug abuse—a major health threat to children. A survey of two thousand teens and one thousand parents by The National Center on Addiction and Substance Abuse at Columbia University (CASA) showed that the safest teens "are those living in two-parent homes who have a positive relationship with both parents, go to both parents equally when they have important decisions to make, have discussed illegal drugs with both parents and report their mom and dad are equally demanding of the teen in terms of grades, homework and personal behavior." Positive health outcomes such as these are the result of moms and dads who are willing to build a strong marriage and home life that will provide the setting for nurturing their children.

Dose of Wisdom

Parent power is key. When there are two parents in the home—and even when one is physically absent—both mom and dad need to be engaged in their child's life. Parents have enormous power over a child's well-being but too many fail to appreciate and use this power.

Joseph A. Califano,
former U.S. Secretary of Health, Education, and Welfare

The need for commitment to marriage and family cannot be overemphasized to parents who desire to raise highly healthy children. Yet no one has a perfect marriage. Some marriages are very unhappy and difficult. So how do you know if it's healthier for your children if you stick it out and try to repair a difficult marriage or if you bail out? It's an agonizingly difficult question for which a parent must carefully weigh the pros and cons.

A recent large-scale, long-term study suggested some answers to the troubling question of what is most healthy for children caught in a difficult marriage. This study clearly demonstrated that the parents' marital unhappiness and discord have a broad negative impact on virtually every dimension of their children's well-being. However, so does a divorce. To better understand the health implications of a poor marriage or a divorce, the researchers examined the negative impacts on children more closely. Their findings were remarkable—and maybe a bit surprising to you.

The researchers discovered that it was only the children in extremely high-conflict homes who benefited when divorce removed conflict from the home. In lower-conflict marriages that ended in divorce—and the study found that perhaps as many as two-thirds of the divorces were of this type—the health of the children nearly always became much worse following divorce. Based on this and other studies, except in the minority of high-conflict marriages, it is almost always better for the children's health if their parents stay together and work out their problems than if they divorce. It is interesting to note that other long-term research suggests that staying in a marriage is generally better for parents as well. These findings reinforce in my mind the devastating impact of divorce on the health of children and their parents.

When it comes to raising healthy children, there simply is no substitute for the parental team. As parents, we would be wise to do everything possible to preserve what is good in our marriages, to build stronger marriages, and to make sacrifices for a home life that nurtures healthy children. But there's more. Each parent as an individual influences a child's health as well. Regardless of the health of our marriage, each parent brings personal qualities and skills to the parenting task. So we would do well to recognize our individual influence on our children's health and develop the skills and attributes that will nurture highly healthy children.

THE ATTRIBUTES OF GREAT PARENTS

No matter what your circumstances are, you can, for the benefit of your children, work to develop the personal attributes of a great parent. The more your children are at risk, the more significant your efforts need to be. If you are an eighty-hour-a-week working dad, a sixty-hour-a-week working mom, a single parent, or a parent of a blended family, the odds are against your children becoming as highly healthy as they could be—*unless* you take action to reduce the risks. Let me share how one dad did this.

When his wife left him for another man, David was wise enough to realize that what his daughter needed most was a dad—not great vacations and lots of "stuff." So David left his business, which had required lots of travel and long hours, and got a job as a high school teacher. The change reduced his income dramatically, but it enabled him to take his daughter to school and pick her up at the end of the day, and it gave him vacation time when she had vacation. He considered all of these things to be crucial to his daughter's well-being. He also created opportunities for his daughter to form mentoring relationships with a few women who reflected the virtues and values David considered to be important. All these actions made a positive difference in his daughter's life and helped her grow up to be a highly healthy young woman.

I knew about the changes David had made to nurture his daughter's health, but quite by accident I learned how personally committed he was to being a dad who modeled virtuous character. I had taken my children out for a meal, and as we were eating I happened to hear parts of a conversation behind me. A teenage girl was asking her father why her mother had left him for another man. Although she was making some judgmental comments about her mother, the father concentrated his comments on the mother's positive points. "What you say is true," he would say. "What she did wasn't right, but I remember when I first met her . . ." and he went on to say something positive. He refused to berate his ex-wife. When I turned around to leave the restaurant, I saw that the father was David.

Great Parents Teach and Model Virtues

In our culture, virtues are often easily overlooked, but it hasn't always been that way. In ancient Rome, parents taught and citizens were encouraged to develop "the personal virtues," the heart of the *Via Romana*—the Roman Way. These virtues were said to have given the Roman Republic the moral strength to conquer and civilize the world. Some historians believe that a widespread decline in these virtues led to the fall of the Roman Empire. Even a quick reading of these virtues reveals how anyone who practices them—adult or child—will be a highly healthy individual:

- *Auctoritas:* Spiritual Authority—the sense of one's social standing, built up through experience, *Pietas,* and *Industria*
- *Comitas:* Humor—ease of manner, courtesy, openness, and friendliness
- *Clementia:* Mercy—mildness and gentleness
- *Dignitas:* Dignity—a sense of self-worth, personal pride
- *Firmitas:* Tenacity—strength of mind, the ability to stick to one's purpose
- *Frugalitas:* Frugalness—economy and simplicity of style, without being miserly
- *Gravitas:* Gravity—a sense of the importance of the matter at hand, responsibility and earnestness
- *Honestas:* Respectability—the image that one presents as a respectable member of society
- *Humanitas:* Humanity—refinement, civilization, learning, and being cultured
- *Industria:* Industriousness—hard work
- *Pietas:* Dutifulness—more than religious piety; a respect for the natural order socially, politically, and religiously (includes the ideas of patriotism and devotion to others)
- *Prudentia:* Prudence—foresight, wisdom, and personal discretion
- *Salubritas:* Wholesomeness—health and cleanliness
- *Severitas:* Sternness—gravity, self-control
- *Veritas*: Truthfulness—honesty in dealing with others

If the Latin virtues feel a bit intimidating, we can count on Benjamin Franklin to simplify things for us. He defined a virtue as simply a "good habit." All of us have habits, which are the ways we behave over and over again. Franklin realized that one of the keys to a rich and satisfying life is to understand which habits are worth developing and which we should eliminate. He also recognized that the development of virtues was a deliberate, lifelong process—not one that ends after reaching adulthood. Franklin committed himself to developing one virtue at a time, and he conducted a daily self-examination to determine what he needed to do to improve.

Dose of Wisdom

TEMPERANCE: Eat not to dullness; drink not to elevation.

SILENCE: Speak not but what may benefit others or yourself; avoid trifling conversation.

ORDER: Let all your things have their places; let each part of your business have its time.

RESOLUTION: Resolve to perform what you ought; perform without fail what you resolve.

FRUGALITY: Make no expense but to do good to others or yourself; that is, waste nothing.

INDUSTRY: Lose no time; be always employed in something useful; cut off all unnecessary actions.

SINCERITY: Use no hurtful deceit; think innocently and justly, and, if you speak, speak accordingly.

JUSTICE: Wrong none by doing injuries, or omitting the benefits that are your duty.

MODERATION: Avoid extremes; forbear resenting injuries so much as you think they deserve.

CLEANLINESS: Tolerate no uncleanliness in body, clothes, or habitation.

TRANQUILITY: Be not disturbed at trifles, or at accidents common or unavoidable.

CHASTITY: Rarely use venery but for health or offspring, never to dullness, weakness, or the injury of your own or another's peace or reputation.

HUMILITY: Imitate Jesus and Socrates.

*Ben Franklin's personal list of virtues
and practical application of each*

In yet another description of virtues, the apostle Paul, a Roman citizen and rabbi who knew well the teachings of Jesus, the Jews, and the Romans, condensed the known virtues into what he called spiritual fruit: "love, joy, peace, patience, kindness, goodness, faithfulness, gentleness, and self-control."

No matter which list of virtues parents prefer, they want their children to practice virtues. The virtues that parents in one survey rated the highest and considered to be essential to teach to their children were honesty and truthfulness

(91 percent), courteousness and politeness (84 percent), self-control and self-discipline (83 percent), and doing their best in school (82 percent). Other virtues these parents said were important to teach children included being independent (74 percent), being frugal (70 percent), having good nutrition and eating habits (68 percent), helping those who are less fortunate (62 percent), and having a strong religious faith (61 percent).

Despite the fact that parents believe teaching virtues is essential to our children's well-being, it isn't something we find easy to do. Americans admit a widespread failure to teach children the essential virtues. And it may be that our failure to teach our children these virtues has had a great impact on the moral health of our nation. A 2000 Harris poll indicated that only 19 percent of Americans hold a positive view of America's morals and values, and a 2001 Barna Research Group survey showed 74 percent of adults expressing concern about the moral condition of the United States.

So how do we think virtues should be taught? Some would say we should do it in our schools. In one survey conducted in 1993, 90 to 97 percent of those surveyed believe public schools should teach virtues such as honesty, democracy, acceptance of different races and ethnic backgrounds, love of country, caring for friends and family members, moral courage, and the Golden Rule. While I agree it is important for schools to teach virtues, and some school systems are beginning to implement such training, teaching virtues is first and foremost the job of parents.

The teaching of virtues is an area in which the parents' individual attributes are essential. Virtues are more effectively caught than taught. Children are most likely to develop the virtues their parents model. When children see their parents working hard alongside them, they learn the virtues of discipline, industry, and tenacity. When children see their parents handle emotionally charged situations with patience, humility, gentleness, and kindness, they learn how to respond in kind. When parents practice justice and respect, children learn to value these virtues. Children best learn from their parents that virtues are both valuable and essential, which motivates them to make the effort to learn and practice them.

Parents are surprisingly candid in admitting their failure to teach the virtues they'd like their children to learn. According to one national survey, parents reported the most difficult virtue to teach is self-control or self-discipline. Only 34 percent of parents feel they've succeeded in this area, while 83 percent feel it's essential to do so—a forty-nine-point gap. The second most difficult area is teaching children to save money and spend it carefully. Only

28 percent of parents think they have succeeded, while 70 percent feel it is essential—a forty-two-point gap. Parents also reported difficulties in teaching independence (a thirty-six-point gap), honesty (a thirty-six-point gap), and eating well (a twenty-eight-point gap). Parents who want to raise highly healthy children will make every effort to close the gap and pass on to their children the virtues they value. They will seek to develop virtues and strengthen their own character while modeling and teaching these virtues to their children. Let me share an example. Barb and I believed it was very important for our children not to lie. It was something we consciously taught them and expected them to practice. If they chose to lie, they faced very specific consequences. Dinnertime was also very important to us, and we typically didn't let the phone interrupt our mealtime together. At times Kate or Scott would answer the phone just as we were preparing for dinner, and I'd say, "Tell them I'm not here."

So one night Scott came to the table and asked, "Why do you make me lie?"

Ouch! My objective in guarding our family time was commendable, but I was asking my son to lie—and that was wrong. We talked about the issue, and I admitted that I had been absolutely wrong and thanked Scott for pointing it out to me. That night we all learned more about what is required to turn our values into virtues.

Of course virtues are taught by instruction as well as by example, and some good tools are available to help children learn. A new PBS series based on William Bennett's *The Book of Virtues* has been growing in popularity. We used the *Character Sketches* material published by the Institute in Basic Youth Conflicts (go to www.highlyhealthy.net to locate these resources). Although Kate and Scott are now in their twenties, they still, in appropriate situations, spontaneously quote lines from these lessons. A number of character education curriculums are available through bookstores and the Internet. Find one, read it, and then begin practicing! This will be an important step toward teaching virtues to your children.

Great Parents Develop Their Parenting Skills

Many parents I observed during my twenty-plus years of delivering babies and caring for families made the mistake of assuming that parenting skills would just happen. The fact is, many of the skills parents need in order to raise highly healthy children are learned, not natural. Highly healthy parents will teach and pass on these skills to their children. If you weren't taught or didn't learn these skills, I suggest you (1) commit to learning and improving your parenting skills and (2) find a mentor to help you develop parenting skills and hold you accountable.

Elizabeth Pantley, author of *Perfect Parenting,* offers four broad approaches for positive parenting that we each can learn and put into practice. She says positive parenting is based on

- action rather than reaction;
- knowledge rather than chance;
- thoughtfulness rather than anger; and
- common sense rather than nonsense.

We can also study and understand the normal development stages of children so we can distinguish "normal" behaviors from "problems." Learning and developing thoughtful approaches to child guidance and discipline is a much better strategy than reacting in anger or resorting to manipulation.

To illustrate the importance of learning good parenting skills, let me tell you about a mom and a dad who each learned parenting skills that changed how they were able to relate to their children. The mom had grown weary of—and even a bit irritated by—reading the same story multiple times to her toddler at bedtime. In a parenting class, the mom learned that every time she reads the same story to her little girl, a different part of the girl's brain will develop. The mom was amazed to find that out, and now she gladly reads the story over and over. This one piece of knowledge helped her stimulate—not stifle—her child's development.

The dad wanted very much to manage his strong-willed son but was afraid he might break the little guy's spirit. When his wife dragged him to a parenting class at their church, he finally learned the difference between breaking the spirit and shaping the will of his son. He had correctly assumed that he could easily damage his son's fragile spirit. But he also learned that a child's will can be made of steel and that confronting willful disobedience yields lifelong benefits. The dad began learning ways to respond to his son that protect his spirit and tame his rebellious nature.

A wide variety of programs have been shown to reduce strife, improve communication, broaden parenting skills, increase stability, and enhance marital happiness—all of which will enhance a child's health. Studies have demonstrated that marriage enrichment and parenting programs are effective and make the case that marriages and parents can do more than merely survive—they can thrive. However, it requires parents who are willing to learn the necessary skills to make their marriage work and who are willing to learn how to become great parents.

Great Parents Invest Their Time and Treasure Wisely

Parents must choose the best ways to invest their time and their treasure (money and things) in their marriage and in their children. Those who choose not to invest wisely will negatively affect the health of their children, their grandchildren, and their great-grandchildren!

The advertising gurus on Madison Avenue in New York City would have us believe that the more things we buy our children, the more secure they will be. Many parents have fallen into the "more is better" and "the best is all that counts" mentality. Yet overindulging our children is *not* essential to their health or well-being; it may, in fact, harm them. Overindulging our children financially is a bit like the classic mistake first-time gardeners make by overwatering plants. Although the right amount of water is necessary and good, too much water will kill a plant.

Parents who overinvest in giving their treasure will often make the mistake of underinvesting in giving their time. For example, many parents will sacrifice spending time with their children (by working two jobs, or having both spouses work) in order to spend more of their precious time at work to provide more treasure that will not contribute to their children's health. According to one national survey, almost half of all parents say their children's "fashion demands" have forced them to sacrifice a family vacation. What is truly tragic is that 25 percent of children surveyed listed a family vacation as one of the top three ways to spend quality time with their parents, while only 11 percent of parents thought so. In other words, parents were willing to keep from their children what they wanted and needed (quality time with their parents) in order to provide frills their children know they don't need.

Dose of Wisdom

The best inheritance a parent can give to his children is a few minutes of his time each day.

Orlando A. Battista, Canadian-American chemist

The mistake of overindulging our children with treasure and robbing them of our time is further demonstrated by the more than 20 percent of parents who admit to having failed to pay bills so they could buy their child's latest craze. Children ages eleven to fifteen were found to be the most demanding, and mothers were most likely to go without (about 58 percent said they had given up buying themselves clothes and 28 percent had sacrificed beauty items such as haircuts). When one realizes that 47 percent of sixteen- to eighteen-year-olds still throw tantrums to get their way, the pressure is understandable. This pressure has left 44 percent of the parents polled unable to save for the future.

Child psychologist Richard Woolfson sees a need for balance: "Parents ... make sacrifices themselves to put a smile on children's faces. That's very positive, but it is important for each parent to help their children understand the processes in making such decisions about purchases." He warned that parents should not take self-sacrifice to extremes because they may end up resenting the child—and the child the parent. Furthermore, overindulging prevents children from learning essential truths about life. He adds, "No matter how many consumer sacrifices a parent willingly makes for their child, children still need to accept that there are limits and that part of family life involves thinking about others."

Many parents have the delusion (a fixed false belief) that treasure is more influential in shaping children than time. But the simple truth is that children internalize, value, and model the virtues of the people they most respect and with whom they spend their time. So parents who spend generous amounts of time with their children have the greatest opportunity to influence and shape their children's lives. Time with your children builds the foundation of an intimate, secure, and irreplaceable relationship with them. It provides an excellent foundation for their future emotional, relational, and spiritual health.

More than the material things that a sixty-hour workweek or a second income may be able to buy, children need generous amounts of time with each of their parents on a regular basis. Some parents think they can give quality time without large quantities of time, but it is impossible to schedule "quality" time. Children share what's on their mind when it comes to mind—which is why quality moments typically occur during quantity time. In addition, children experience many small events each day that have an impact on them. So parents who spend generous amounts of time with their children are best able to understand and address their fears, hesitations, and actions.

Distinguished child development expert Mary Ainsworth observes: "It's very hard to become a sensitively responsive mother if you're away from your child 10 hours a day." And, contrary to what many parents believe, the need for appropriate and strong attachments with parents doesn't go away as a child grows older. The National Longitudinal Study of Adolescent Health, a survey of 90,000 seventh through twelfth graders released in 1997, revealed that adolescents with strong emotional attachments to their parents and teachers are much less likely to use drugs and alcohol, attempt suicide, engage in violence, or become sexually active at an early age.

Even so, I've still had parents declare they were going to strive for quality time with their children due to the fact they were unwilling to make the lifestyle changes that would allow them to invest in quantity time with their children. The founder and chairman of the board at Focus on the Family and internationally recognized child psychology expert, Dr. James Dobson, doesn't buy into the myth of having to choose between the virtues of quantity and quality. "We won't accept that forced choice in any other area of our lives," he observes, "so why is it only relevant to our children?" Dr. Dobson goes on to illustrate his point:

> Let's suppose you've looked forward all day to eating at one of the finest restaurants in town. The waiter brings you a menu, and you order the most expensive steak in the house. But when the meal arrives, you see a tiny piece of meat about one-inch square in the center of the plate. When you complain about the size of the steak, the waiter says, "Sir, I recognize that the portion is small, but that's the finest corn-fed beef money can buy. You'll never find a better bite of meat than we've served you tonight. As to the portion, I hope you understand that it's not the quantity that matters, it's the quality that counts." You would object, and for good reason. Why? Because both quality and quantity are important in many areas of our lives, including how we relate to children. They need our time and the best we have to give them.

To develop stronger, healthier relationships, say the authors of a study conducted by the Atlanta-based Boys & Girls Clubs of America, requires that parents give their children time and involve themselves in activities their children enjoy. "Kids are saying that they want the activities to be more fun-focused, more interactive," said Roxanne Spillett, the organization's president. "Fun is an essential ingredient."

The findings of this study—the result of one thousand telephone interviews with parents and children in the same families—document patterns I noticed in my practice for years. Fifty-two percent of parents admit they don't spend enough quality time with their children, and 57 percent of children believe their parents' work gets in the way of meaningful time. Virtually any time parents and kids spend together is good time. But if you choose to try to give your children quality time without quantity time, you may end up providing neither.

THE TEN COMMITMENTS OF GREAT PARENTS

Before I conclude this chapter, I want to share my adaptation of the ten commitments of great parents developed by psychologist Todd E. Linaman. These commitments, which I'll explore further in subsequent chapters, remind us of the most important sacrifices we parents can make to raise highly healthy children. These commitments (with perhaps the exception of number 7) are choices each of us can make, regardless of our personal life circumstances.

1. *Provide for physical needs.* Growing children need healthy diets, adequate clothing, quality health care, and protection from harm.
2. *Be there for them.* When your children talk to you, turn off the television, face them, and *really* listen. As much as possible, attend Little League games, school conferences, and band concerts. Your presence, attention, and availability will make a significant difference in the lives of your children.
3. *Give them "roots and wings."* Children need to try new things. They need the opportunity to try and to learn from the experience. Supportive family "roots" will soften any falls and give them a stable place to land.
4. *Balance individuality with absolutes.* Each child is unique. Celebrate individual strengths and try to see life from your child's perspective. Show respect for personal preferences and fears. At the same time, operate from the strength of your convictions. Children need the security of unmovable boundaries and guidelines for behavior.
5. *Hold them accountable.* Children want to do what's right, and they want to be accepted. If they've done wrong, encourage them to make amends. Doing so restores their self-respect and lets them know that their behaviors have consequences.
6. *Admit when you're wrong.* As parents we make mistakes, and our children can see it—whether we admit it or not. If we're willing

to say, "I blew it; I'm sorry," our children learn that our relationship with them is more important than maintaining the upper
hand. It gives them the freedom to admit their mistakes as well.
Facing the truth is a key to good emotional health.

7. *Love your spouse.* Your children need the security and example of
   your love for one another.

8. *Practice what you preach.* Actions speak louder than words. If you
   tell your children to respect their teachers while you bad-mouth
   your boss, don't expect good behavior reports at school conference time! Fight the temptation to just drop them off at church—
   go with them!

9. *Demonstrate a love of learning.* If you read for enjoyment and self-
   improvement, your children are more likely to enjoy learning.
   Read with them and discuss new ideas to stimulate their thinking. Help your children reach conclusions for themselves. Also,
   expose your children to new opportunities for learning, such as
   going to the library, surfing the Internet with them, and taking
   them to museums.

10. *Never give up on them!* As our children grow up, some of them
    will make us think we have done a good job; others may make us
    wonder if we did anything right at all. The time comes when we
    have to back off and let our children make their own decisions
    and mistakes. But we must never stop loving them or encourag-
    ing them to be the best they can be.

Congratulations! We've covered the basics of what a highly healthy child
is, and we've briefly considered the crucial role parents have—individually
and as a couple—in nurturing healthy children. Now let's begin examining the
essentials of raising a highly healthy child.

PART TWO

The

TEN ESSENTIALS OF NURTURING HIGHLY HEALTHY CHILDREN

Chapter Three

Be Proactive in Preventing Physical Disease

I remember the first time I watched the movie *The Wizard of Oz* with my parents at home. Do you remember the part where Dorothy exclaims, "There's no place like home. There's no place like home"? I was sitting on the floor in front of my dad, and he was rubbing my shoulders. We had just come back from swimming together at the YMCA. I remember thinking, *Yep, there's no place like home!*

The home—the place where children interact with and observe their parents every day—is a child's most important classroom for good health. Whether we like it or not, we parents are powerful models. Our children are designed to look to us as models for thoughts, values, and behavior. They learn more from watching and imitating our actions than they ever learn from our preaching or criticism—both of which can crush their spirit. So parents who model highly healthy preventive health care are more likely to have highly healthy children.

Dose of Wisdom

What is learned in the cradle lasts to the grave.

French proverb

Ensuring good health for our children requires more than good modeling, however. We parents also need to be intentional about good health maintenance and prevention. There are specific things we need to do for our children's health, things we need to teach our children about health, and things we need to monitor in order to keep our children healthy. So let's explore the major steps you can take to prevent physical health problems for your children.

SEE TO IT THAT YOUR CHILDREN RECEIVE REGULAR WELL-CHILD CHECKUPS

Regular well-child checkups are one of the most important ways to give your child a healthy start. A well-child checkup is simply a visit to a child's doctor when the child is *not* sick. My well-child visits with physician Gloria Weir brought a tear to my eye many times. Mom took all four of us boys to Dr. Weir when we were sick and for our checkups. Usually our checkups included a shot, so there were tears going to and coming home from her office. As a young boy, I did not think a loving parent would subject a child to shots, but now I know differently.

Well-child checkups are important because a healthy start during the formative years affects a child's entire life. Well-child visits within the child's first year are particularly important because infants undergo substantial changes in cognitive abilities, physical growth, motor skills, hand-eye coordination, and social and emotional growth. Very young children need regular checkups so their growth and development can be measured and to ensure that they receive immunizations on schedule. Early and periodic screenings, as well as diagnostic tests, are essential to a comprehensive health care program that seeks to prevent illness and disease.

During each visit, your child's doctor should review your child's complete health and developmental histories and conduct a comprehensive physical exam. (Fortunately, most Medicaid and insurance programs now cover the cost of these checkups.) Immunizations or lab work may also be needed. Your child's doctor also has the opportunity to dispense health advice that can help you prevent potential health problems. One of the most valuable parts of the visit is the opportunity you have to ask questions about your child's health. It's always a good idea to write down your questions prior to your appointment so you don't forget them.

Many studies support my recommendation that children receive six well-child visits during the first year of life. Although there are a number of published schedules for well-child visits, here's the schedule I used:

- FIRST YEAR: 2 weeks, 2 months, 4 months, 6 months, 9 months, and 12 months
- SECOND YEAR: 15 months, 18 months, 2 years
- AGES 3–5: 3 years, 4 years, 5 years
- AGES 6–8: at least once but preferably yearly
- AGES 8–11: at least once but preferably yearly

I cannot overemphasize the importance of well-child care. Research shows that many children in the United States do not receive the minimum recommended number of preventive health care visits. In fact, an American Academy of Pediatrics survey showed that more than 23 percent of children did not receive the recommended number of well-child visits during the year prior to the survey.

Most doctors who care for children can recount dozens of instances when preventive exams allowed them to discover serious problems during very early stages. One day, when I was examining the neck of a preschool lad, I was surprised to find a nickel-sized lump. It was rock-hard and didn't move under my fingers like a normal lymph node. The biopsy showed a cancer that was much easier to treat at the early stages. I'm glad to say this little guy is now in college and has been in remission for more than fifteen years.

Resource Box   Helpful Hints

What a Well-Child Visit Should Include

- Height and weight evaluation (with Body Mass Index calculation for age two years and up)
- Age-appropriate developmental screening
- Vision and hearing screenings
- Checking of vital signs, including blood pressure (three years and up)
- Nutritional assessments
- Immunizations
- Laboratory procedures such as urinalysis, tuberculin (TB) skin test, and lead screening (at some visits)
- Advice about preventive measures

SEE TO IT THAT YOUR CHILDREN RECEIVE APPROPRIATE IMMUNIZATIONS

When it comes to protecting children against disease and ill health—which is of prime importance to parents and health professionals—vaccines are widely regarded as one of the most effective ways to prevent many common childhood illnesses. Yet few parents realize or even talk about how essential vaccinations are to their children's health. In fact, many parents in the United States are confused about vaccines. They often do not understand the concept of population immunization and know little about the diseases against which their children are being vaccinated.

I know from talking with parents just how hard it can be to get understandable, accurate information on vaccines. But in order for your children to become highly healthy, you *must* be well-informed. If you know little about vaccinations or are making vaccination-related decisions based on inaccurate information, you risk harming your child. You simply must educate yourself.

Let me share why this is so important. Childhood vaccinations in the United States have dramatically reduced diseases such as whooping cough, mumps, polio, smallpox, diphtheria, tetanus, measles, and chicken pox. Because we have so little experience with these diseases today (smallpox, for example, hasn't been seen for decades), it is easy to forget how serious these illnesses can be.

That's what happened in Great Britain during the 1970s. The vaccination program had been so successful that once-common and potentially fatal infectious diseases such as pertussis (whooping cough), German measles, and polio were rarely, if ever, seen. In fact, the side effects of the vaccines, even though very rare, had become more common than the diseases they were preventing. So increasing numbers of parents refused to vaccinate their children. By the late 1970s, at the time I was in a teaching fellowship at the Queen's Medical Center in Nottingham, England, these diseases were coming back with a vengeance. That's why, during my medical training, I was seeing cases of diseases I only had read about in textbooks—pertussis, diphtheria, mumps, and measles.

The most horrible case I saw took place one night in the "labour ward." A teenage mother, whose parents had never allowed her to be immunized, must have come in contact with the rubella virus early in her pregnancy. The baby girl she delivered had congenital rubella syndrome and was horribly deformed. The baby had cataracts and congenital heart disease. She was blind and deaf. She had a tiny head with evidence of brain damage, an enlarged spleen that kept her blood from clotting properly, and a poorly functioning liver. I had never seen a case like this before and have, thank God, never seen one since.

I still remember the rather stoic attending physician, with misty eyes, shaking his head and saying, "It could have been prevented. It should have been prevented." The baby died a few days later. Her grandparents had to live with the fatal consequences of what they had presumed was a wise decision. Uninformed or inaccurately informed health care decisions are clearly a threat to your children's health.

Unfortunately, some of the most easily accessed information confuses the issue. More than two-thirds of adults in the United States use the Internet to find health-related information. Yet research shows that less than 20 percent of medical information on the Internet is reliable and authoritative according to medical profession standards. Due to the way Internet search engines link websites—which has little or nothing to do with quality—well-meaning but unsuspecting parents searching the Web may be sent first to inaccurate, misleading, or downright false information.

Researchers in 2002 searched the Internet for vaccination advice and concluded there is a high probability that parents will encounter elaborate, inflammatory and highly inaccurate anti-vaccination material. Researchers also found that the content on many sites was biased rhetoric or was scientifically invalid. Because of this, professional medical groups are becoming increasingly concerned about groups that oppose vaccinations and use the Internet to unethically campaign for their cause.

Resource Box   *Helpful Hints*

For a list of Internet sites I consider particularly helpful in raising highly healthy children, visit my website at www.highlyhealthy.net.

So what's the truth about vaccinations? It's really not difficult to understand. At a time when most parents are having their children vaccinated, parents who refuse to vaccinate wrongly think that their children are probably safe without the vaccine and that their refusal does not affect other children. Although the disease may still occur in small numbers, chances are low that any children—vaccinated or not—will get the disease. However, as increasing numbers of parents choose not to vaccinate, everything changes. When vaccination levels fall below 90 percent or so in any given region, parents who do not vaccinate their children put their children and other unvaccinated children at higher risk for the illness. For example, in the United States, unvaccinated children are about twenty-two times as likely to acquire measles and six times as likely to acquire whooping cough as vaccinated children.

Falling vaccination rates, which as of this writing are occurring in many areas of the United States, lend credibility to fears that previously common and now preventable diseases will once again affect our children. In 2002, a dramatic example surfaced in Europe. Consider the facts:

- Fewer than five health care providers opposed to vaccinating children against measles are believed to be responsible for a measles epidemic in the district of Coburg in the German state of Bavaria.
- Coburg has a population of fewer than 100,000 people, but more than 1,100 of them contracted measles in 2002.
- About 90 percent of the cases were in children ages fourteen or younger, and several children required hospitalization.
- Seventy-six percent of children in Coburg had been vaccinated, but at least 90 percent of children in a given population need to be immunized to effectively combat measles epidemics.

The possibility of similar outbreaks of preventable infectious diseases frightens me. Immunizations are essential for highly healthy children.

Resource Box   **Helpful Hints**

Which Immunizations Do My Children Need?

Most childhood immunizations are given during the first two years of life, some within hours of birth. Some preschool programs and virtually all schools require proof of immunization before a child can be admitted to school—unless a child has a physician's exemption. Check with your children's doctor or your local health department to find out which shots they need, or go to my website (www.highly healthy.net), which lists Internet sites that provide the most up-to-date recommendations. Shots for children are also available at most public health clinics, where they are either inexpensive or free.

One immunization many parents don't consider for their children is the annual influenza (flu) shot. Although most of us understand the importance of a yearly flu shot for people ages sixty-five and older and for high-risk children or children with chronic illnesses, many parents overlook the need for flu shots for healthy children—which is unfortunate because most experts believe that flu epidemics begin and spread to adults from younger children. In addition, because young and otherwise healthy children are at increased risk for influenza-related hospitalization, the Centers for Disease Control and Prevention (CDC) and the American Academy of Pediatrics (AAP) now recommend influenza vaccination of healthy children ages six months to twenty-three months. For children over age two, the vaccine is optional. Children ages five and older may receive a nasal spray form of the immunization, thus avoiding an injection.

The Truth about Vaccine Myths

As parents, we're constantly exposed to newspaper articles and television programs that falsely depict the frightening side of vaccines. In these stories the scoundrels are said to be greedy vaccine manufacturers, uninterested physicians, and burdensome regulatory agencies. Perhaps the most dangerous by-product of this reporting—apart from the fact that these stories may lead parents to refuse potentially life-saving vaccines—is that these myths are presented on many misleading antivaccination websites in a manner that seems believable. So I'd like to help you sort through the most common vaccine-related myths, using the well-researched information in an excellent resource titled *Vaccines: What Every Parent Should Know* by Paul A. Offit, M.D. and Louis M. Bell, M.D. As we go along, I'll help you separate fact from fiction.

Myth: Vaccines Don't Work

Probably the best recent example of the positive impact of vaccines is the Hib vaccine, which prevents meningitis, ear infections, and other serious infections caused by the bacterium *Haemophilus influenzae type b* (Hib). When the current Hib vaccine was introduced to this country in 1990, Hib was the most common cause of bacterial meningitis. For decades, Hib had caused approximately 15,000 cases of meningitis and 400 to 500 deaths every year. After the current Hib vaccine was introduced, the incidence of Hib meningitis declined to fewer than fifty cases per year—typical of all widely used vaccines. The incidence of disease is dramatically reduced within several years after a vaccine against a disease is introduced. Not only do vaccines work, they work phenomenally well—and they save lives!

Myth: Vaccines Aren't Necessary

Most parents today have never seen a case of measles, mumps, German measles, polio, diphtheria, tetanus, or whooping cough. Thus it's understandable that some would question the continued need for vaccines. Even if the incidence of disease is low, there are still three important reasons for immunizations:

- Some diseases (such as chicken pox) are still so prevalent in this country that a decision not to be immunized is tantamount to a decision to get this disease.
- Some diseases (such as measles, mumps, German measles, and pertussis) continue to occur, but at fairly low levels. If immunization rates drop, outbreaks of these diseases will again occur, and children will die.
- Some diseases (such as polio and diphtheria) have been virtually eliminated from this country, but outbreaks of these diseases still occur in other countries. Given the high rate of international travel, travelers and immigrants could easily import these diseases (as they did with Severe Acute Respiratory Syndrome [SARS] in 2003).

Myth: Vaccines Are Unsafe

Despite what is often falsely reported in the media, all recommended vaccines are extraordinarily safe. When you consider that the 3.5 to 4 million children born every year in the United States receive more than twenty different vaccines to protect them from at least eleven different preventable diseases by the time they are six years old, and that some of these vaccines have existed for more than fifty years, I think you'll agree that the record of vaccine safety in this country is remarkable.

For the most part, vaccine side effects are usually limited to pain and tenderness where the shot was given or to low-grade fever. But worry persists because of some problems that occurred with the "old" pertussis vaccine and the "old" oral polio vaccine (OPV)—problems that have been remedied.

The old pertussis vaccine (the preparation called DTP, which stopped being recommended for use in the United States in 1997) rarely caused temporary seizures, persistent crying, and high fever, but no permanent damage. Parents understandably found it difficult to watch their children suffer these side effects. The new pertussis vaccine (DTaP, approved by the FDA in 1991) is purer than the old vaccine and almost completely eliminates these rare side effects.

Because it was a live vaccine, the OPV (oral polio vaccine) caused—but very, very rarely—complete and lifelong paralysis, usually after the first dose. Because the wild poliovirus was eliminated from the Western Hemisphere in 1991, the only children who now get polio in this country are those who received OPV. Therefore, in 2000, the CDC recommended discontinuation of OPV, to be replaced with four doses of inactivated polio vaccine (IPV), which has not been shown to cause paralysis, but does have to be given by injection.

Myth: Infants Are Too Young to Get Vaccinated

It's very important to make sure that infants are fully immunized against certain diseases by the age of six months. Children need to be immunized during the first few months of life because a number of vaccine-preventable diseases could otherwise infect them. Fortunately, young infants are surprisingly good at building immunity to viruses and bacteria. About 95 percent of children given DTaP, Hib, and hepatitis B virus vaccines will be fully protected by six months of age.

Some of the diseases for which young infants need protection include pertussis, Hib meningitis, and hepatitis. Consider these facts:

- Pertussis (whooping cough) infects about seven thousand children and causes six deaths every year in the United States. Almost all of the cases occur in nonimmunized children less than one year of age.
- Unvaccinated children under two years old are five hundred times more likely to catch Hib meningitis than an immunized child if someone with an Hib infection is living in the home.
- About 90 percent of newborns whose mothers are infected with hepatitis B will contract hepatitis and go on to develop chronic liver disease, cirrhosis, and possibly liver cancer. Some will die.

Myth: It's Better to Be Naturally Infected Than Immunized

It is true that natural infection almost always causes better immunity than vaccination. In fact, only the Hib and tetanus vaccines are better at inducing immunity than natural infection. Natural infection causes immunity after just one infection, but vaccines usually create immunity only after several doses over a period of time. For example, DTaP, hepatitis B, and polio vaccines are each recommended at least three times during the first six months of life.

The difference lies in the price paid for immunity. The price paid for vaccination is the inconvenience of several shots and an occasional sore injection site. The price paid for a single natural infection may be paralysis from natural polio infection, mental retardation or hearing difficulties from natural Hib infection, liver failure or death from natural hepatitis B infection, deafness from natural mumps infection, or pneumonia from natural varicella infection. Which price do you want your child to pay for immunity?

Myth: Vaccines Weaken the Immune System

Natural infection with certain viruses can weaken the immune system. So when children are infected with one virus, they can't fight off other viruses or bacteria as easily. This happens most notably during natural infection with chicken pox or measles. Children infected with chicken pox are susceptible to certain bacterial infections (flesh-eating bacteria, for example). Children infected with measles are more susceptible to bacterial infections (resulting in sepsis) of the bloodstream.

But vaccines are different. The viruses in the measles and chicken pox vaccines (the so-called vaccine viruses) are very different from those that cause measles and chicken pox infections (the wild-type viruses). Vaccine viruses cannot weaken the immune system.

Myth: Vaccines Cause Autism

In 1998, a study published in the English journal *Lancet* reported that autism might be caused by the combination measles, mumps, and rubella (MMR) vaccine. The report claimed that children given this vaccine developed intestinal inflammation that preceded the development of autism. In response, the Medical Research Council of Britain set up a panel to investigate a possible link between MMR vaccine and autism. A subsequent study showed that there was no association between vaccines and autism.

Since then, a number of large studies in several countries have shown no association between the MMR vaccine and autism. Medical organizations such as the American Academy of Pediatrics, the Centers for Disease Control and Prevention, the American Academy of Family Physicians, the Institute of Medicine, and the Advisory Committee on Immunization Practices to the CDC, which are composed of scientists, clinicians, epidemiologists, parents, and statisticians, have all concluded there is no link. If well-controlled, adequately analyzed studies clearly showed that MMR caused or could cause autism, experts in the field would quickly ask for the vaccine to be withdrawn.

Myth: A Preservative Contained in Many Vaccines Harms Children

In 1999, a study revealed that the preservative thimerosal, a mercury-containing compound present in many vaccines, caused several infants to have levels of mercury in their blood that exceeded guidelines recommended by the Environmental Protection Agency (EPA). (Preservatives are used in vaccines to reduce the risk of contamination by bacteria once the vial is opened.) Exposure to high levels of mercury, especially in the developing child before birth, is associated with neurological disturbances. When this study was first described, physicians, scientists, and public health officials quickly assessed the situation and found that

- the levels of mercury did not exceed guidelines recommended by the Food and Drug Administration (FDA), the agency responsible for the safety of drugs and biologics (such as vaccines);
- vaccines containing thimerosal have been used since the 1930s, and no child has ever been proven to have been harmed by trace amounts of thimerosal in vaccines;
- thimerosal contains ethyl mercury, not methyl mercury (the most harmful form of mercury); and
- mercury is eliminated from the body within two months, an interval commonly used to administer vaccines.

Even though the FDA and CDC concluded that thimerosal was safe for infants, they feared that vaccines containing thimerosal would be perceived as unsafe by the public. Therefore, in 1999, the CDC recommended that thimerosal be removed from vaccines as quickly and efficiently as possible. Today, all vaccines on the recommended childhood immunization schedule appear in either a thimerosal-free form or a form of thimerosal that is reduced by greater than 95 percent.

Myth: Vaccine-Preventable Diseases Occur More Often in Vaccinated People Than in Unvaccinated People

Superficially speaking, this statement is true. However, it is important to understand why. Medical doctors Paul Offit and Louis Bell explain:

> Let's say that among 100 young adults living in a college dormitory, 95 were vaccinated against measles and 5 were not. An outbreak of measles then strikes. Six of the 95 vaccinated people get measles, as do 4 of the 5 unvaccinated ones. This would seem to indicate that vaccinated people get measles more commonly than unvaccinated people. But let's look more critically. The attack rate for measles in the unvaccinated group was 80 percent (4 of 5), whereas the attack rate for vaccinated people was only 6 percent (6 of 95). So people were much less likely to get measles if they received the measles vaccine.

A study recently reported in the *Journal of the American Medical Association* found that unvaccinated people were thirty-five times as likely to get measles as vaccinated people.

Myth: Vaccines, If Administered during the First Two Years of Life, Can Cause Diabetes.

One researcher claimed that infants immunized with one dose of Hib vaccine at twenty-four months of age were less likely to get diabetes than if they received four doses of the Hib vaccine (at three, four, six, and eighteen months of age). He concluded that the risk of diabetes could be reduced if children did not receive vaccines at a young age.

After carefully reviewing the data, researchers discovered that analytic methods used in the study were incorrect. A ten-year follow-up study showed that the incidence of diabetes was the same in those who had been immunized early and those who were immunized later. No evidence exists to support the notion that vaccines should be delayed.

Myth: The DTP Vaccine Caused Deafness in the 1994 Miss America Beauty Pageant Winner

The Miss America winner was reputed to have become permanently deaf because of a bad DTP vaccine, but this story was totally false. Her deafness occurred after she contracted bacterial meningitis caused by Haemophilus influenzae type b (Hib), a bacterium for which a vaccine has since become available. Fortunately, the Hib vaccine has virtually eliminated Hib meningitis and its resulting deafness.

Myth: The Polio Virus Vaccine Is Contaminated with a Virus That Causes Cancer

Early batches of poliovirus vaccine used in the late 1950s and early 1960s were contaminated with a monkey virus called Simian Virus 40, or SV40. Recently an investigator found proteins made by SV40 virus in unusual tumors in adults. The studies were suggestive enough that the National Institutes of Health continued to research the association. However, subsequent studies have *not* confirmed the initial observation. No currently manufactured polio vaccines contain SV40, so current poliovirus vaccines pose no risk of ill effects from the virus.

Resource Box   *Helpful Hints*

There are many more myths related to vaccines. For additional information on the myths I've explained and clarification of more vaccine myths, check my website at www.highlyhealthy.net.

There are also moral and ethical issues surrounding the use of some vaccines. One of the most disturbing is the use of tissues from unborn children to prepare certain vaccines. You can find this information in the appendix (pages 297–98).

PREVENTIVE DENTAL CARE

Although this topic may have come as a surprise to you—it certainly did to most parents I dealt with in my practice—preventive dental care for children, even young children, is very important. Early dental intervention is relatively easy and effective. Without preventive dental care, more than 50 percent of children have detectable tooth decay (dental caries or cavities) by middle childhood, and by late adolescence about 80 percent of children have acquired this preventable infectious disease.

Childhood oral disease has significant medical and financial consequences. If the prospect of bad teeth, cavities, and bad breath isn't enough to keep your children brushing, a report released in May 2000 by the U.S. Surgeon General provides a new incentive: poor oral health contributes to other serious health problems, such as diabetes and heart disease. The report also indicated that poor oral health can contribute to lung disease, stroke, and low birth weight. Yet nearly half of the children in a recent survey did not receive the American Academy of Pediatric Dentistry's minimal recommendation of two annual dental visits, and 21 percent of all children did not even have a single dental visit during the previous year. Very young children were the least likely to receive dental care.

The American Academy of Pediatrics (AAP) recommends that by six months of age, all babies—even though they have few or no teeth at this age—should be assessed by a physician or dentist to determine their risk of developing tooth decay. Children who appear most likely to develop cavities should have their first visit with a dentist before the recommended age of twelve months.

In addition to regular dental checkups, parents need to ensure that their children learn and practice daily oral hygiene. Good oral hygiene and eating habits can help reduce cavities, but in recent history the use of fluoride has dramatically reduced tooth decay and cavities. Medical and dental research has proven that fluoride reduces cavities in children and adults, helps prevent tooth decay, and can even repair early stages of tooth decay. For that reason, fluoride is added to our water, mouth rinses, and toothpaste.

Unfortunately, many parents are misinformed about fluoride and fluoridation. Fluoride, a mineral that occurs naturally in virtually all water sources, comes from the element fluorine—the seventeenth most abundant element in the earth's crust. Fluoride, like any nutrient, is safe and effective when used appropriately and in the proper amount. Community water fluoridation, which has been practiced for more than fifty years, is simply the process of adjusting the fluoride content of the local water supply to the recommended level for optimal dental health, a practice that has proved to reduce decay in both children and adults.

Fluoride can be applied in either systemic (water fluoridation or dietary supplements) or topical (toothpaste, mouth rinse professionally applied) preparations. The American Dental Association reminds parents that the effective prevention of dental decay requires "the proper mix of both forms of fluoride (topical and systemic)." So let's consider the benefits of each.

Topical fluorides strengthen teeth, making them more decay-resistant. The most common method of "self-applied fluoride" is the use of a fluoride-containing toothpaste. The American Dental Association recommends that children (over two years of age) and adults use a fluoride-containing toothpaste displaying the ADA Seal of Acceptance.

However, caution is in order. It can be harmful if a child uses and swallows too much toothpaste. For this reason, and because young children tend not to brush their teeth very well, most pediatric dentists recommend that parents apply only a pea-sized dab of toothpaste to the brush and then brush the child's teeth for them. When the parents (or dentist) are convinced the child is brushing correctly, the child may do this on his or her own.

Systemic fluorides are ingested into the body and are incorporated into tooth structures from the inside out. Systemic fluorides also give topical protection because the fluoride is then present in saliva, which continually bathes the teeth. Although community water fluoridation is an extremely effective and inexpensive means of obtaining the fluoride necessary for optimal tooth decay prevention, not everyone lives in a community with a fluoridated water source, and most home water filters remove fluoride from the water. For those children ages six months to sixteen years, fluoride is available in prescription-only tablets, drops, or lozenges. Your child's dentist or physician can prescribe the correct dosage.

WHEN IS IT TIME TO CALL THE DOCTOR?

Although "an ounce of prevention is worth a pound of cure," there are many times when no amount of prevention will keep our children from being sick or injured. When this happens, what do you do? How much treatment do you try to apply at home? When do you need to call the doctor's office? When do you need to take a child in for a visit? In my practice these were some of the most frequently asked questions by parents—especially new parents.

Caring for children is a learning process, and parents need to learn when to call the doctor and when not to. In our medical office, we told parents to call our staff for help whenever they were concerned about their child's health or well-being and didn't know what to do. By talking with your child's health care professionals, you will learn about his or her routine care as well as how to handle common problems and illnesses. It is essential for your child's doctor to encourage your questions and provide an atmosphere in which you feel comfortable asking any question. As you gain more experience—and the confidence that goes with it—you'll find that you need to call less often.

Never underestimate your parental instincts, especially if you are a mom. Parents almost always know their children best. They're much more likely to know when something isn't right before it's obvious to someone else—even to your child's doctor. So the rule in my medical practice was this: If *you* are concerned, you need to call your child's doctor or nurse. Most parents have no medical training. Some problems that may seem serious to you as a parent wouldn't concern me as a physician. On the other side of the coin, you may think that something is trivial when it's really an important sign of a health problem. You learn the difference by calling your child's doctor or nurse.

Some minor illnesses, conditions, and injuries can be treated at home, but your child will, at some point, exhibit symptoms that require medical attention. I've provided a detailed list of symptoms and how you should respond to them in appendix 1 (page 293). For more general guidelines, you should call your child's doctor if you notice changes in your child's behavior or activity level, or if you observe other symptoms that worry you. When you call, be prepared to describe your child's symptoms and behavior to the doctor.

Resource Box   ***Helpful Hints***

Symptoms That Need Attention

You should respond quickly to any of the following symptoms:

- Changes in color (paleness or bluish color around the lips, face, and nails; yellowish skin or eyes)
- Body becomes unusually floppy or stiff
- One eye (or both) becomes pink, red, or swollen, or leaks sticky fluid
- Red or tender navel
- White patches in the mouth
- Difficulty breathing, swallowing, nursing, eating, or speaking
- Blood in the stools
- Crying for a long time; child can't be comforted
- Refusal to eat
- Unusually cranky or tired

- Chills that make the body shake
- Loses consciousness (child faints, has a seizure, and so on)
- Severe headache
- Nasal fluid is strange color, has a bad smell, or is bloody
- Earache
- Hearing loss
- Blood or fluid coming out of the mouth or ears
- Changes in vision; eyes are hurt by light
- Stiffness or pain in the neck
- Severe sore throat
- Uncontrolled drooling
- Rapid breathing
- Severe cough, cough that brings up blood or that lasts a long time
- Very bad stomach pain
- Swollen stomach
- Pain in the back, pain with urination, frequent urination
- Urine that is a strange color, has a bad smell, or is very dark
- Pain, redness, or swelling around a joint not caused by injury
- Cut or scrape that appears infected (red, oozes pus, tender, swollen, hot)

WHAT ABOUT THE RELATIONAL, EMOTIONAL, AND SPIRITUAL WHEELS?

This entire chapter has focused on a few principles of preventive medicine, at least as they pertain to the physical health wheel. You may be wondering, *What about the other health wheels? Isn't it equally important to prevent problems in the emotional, relational, and spiritual wheels?*

This is a great question, and my answer may surprise you: "No!"

"What?" you may cry out. "Are you nuts? Do you really think the physical wheel is more important than the others?"

I'd smile and reply, "No." As you calm down, I'd explain that the other three wheels are actually *more* important than the physical wheel. Is the physical wheel important? Absolutely. But remember, the physical wheel is the only one of the four that is guaranteed to slowly run down and one day come to a grinding halt. The physical wheel slows down as we age and stops when we die. However, the other three wheels—the emotional, relational, and spiritual wheels—do not stop when we die. They continue eternally. This is why the apostle Paul wrote, "For physical training is of some value, but godliness has value for all things, holding promise for both the present life and the life to come."

Your job as a parent definitely includes preventing physical disease whenever possible, but your role in preventing emotional, relational, and spiritual disease; distress; disorder; and disability is even more important. You see, raising and nurturing children who are highly healthy in these three areas is the job of the family. The healthier your family is in these areas, the more likely it is that your children will be healthy as well.

When there is trouble on the home front, children can suffer physically, but they suffer the most emotionally, socially, and spiritually. A special national commission met in the 1980s to examine the general health of children, especially adolescents. These authorities on child development became so concerned about what they found that their published report was entitled *Code Blue*. They concluded, "Never before has one generation of American adolescents been less healthy, less cared for, or less prepared for life."

Commenting on this report, Dr. James Dobson observes, "This is occurring, mind you, in one of the most affluent and privileged nations in the history of the world. It is a direct result of marital disintegration and related forces at work against the family." Dr. Dobson concludes that even when families are intact, the research clearly points out that our children are highly unlikely to become healthy emotionally, relationally, and spiritually because we—their parents—are "distracted, overworked, harassed, exhausted, disinterested, chemically dependent, divorced, or simply unable to cope."

So, yes, preserving and enhancing your child's physical health is essential, but I'll spend much more time sharing how you can concentrate your time, efforts, and prayers in building up and protecting your child's emotional, relational and spiritual health.

Chapter Four

Build Your Child's Health Care Team

Tonya brought five-year-old Abby to my office to be evaluated for fever and listlessness. "Dr. Larimore, I think she has meningitis."

I wasn't alarmed. First-time moms like Tonya can become concerned over minor illnesses, so I carefully examined Abby. She seemed alert, had no neck stiffness, and absolutely no sign of infection. *I don't think she has meningitis,* I thought.

"Tonya, I think it's probably just a virus."

"But I'm worried," she responded honestly.

I explained why I didn't think Abby had meningitis, but Tonya was not to be dissuaded. "I hear what you're saying, Doctor. I'm just worried that it's meningitis."

I understood her concern. Meningitis is an infection of the lining of the brain and spinal cord that results in fever, stiff neck, listlessness, and sometimes a rash. The most dangerous of these infections can be fatal if not treated quickly. Having learned to value and honor a mother's intuition, I said, "God has given a mother's intuition only to mothers." I then explained that if Tonya wanted to be 100 percent sure, Abby would need a spinal tap. We discussed the risks and benefits of the procedure and the options to treat the fever at home with acetaminophen and fluids. Somewhat reluctantly, but wisely, I thought, Tonya chose the latter course. I asked her to call if she encountered any problem at all.

About three hours later, Tonya called my home, trying to locate me. Barb, my wife, answered the phone. Tonya could barely speak through her trembling lips. "I think Abby's worse. I think her neck is stiff. I can't control the fever. She seems so sleepy." Barb wisely counseled Tonya to take Abby to the emergency room and assured her that I'd meet them there.

Abby still seemed normal when I saw her. Even her white blood cell count was normal. (With infection, it's usually elevated.) Nevertheless, Tonya remained convinced that her daughter was very ill. At her insistence, I did the spinal tap. The fluid looked perfectly normal, but the lab tests were undeniable: Abby had a very early form of Hib bacterial meningitis! (I should point out that this case occurred before the Hib vaccine was available, and it was the last case of invasive Hib infection I saw in my career. Most physicians trained since the onset of the Hib vaccine have not seen cases like this.)

Soon after I admitted her to the hospital, Abby became very sick, and her course of treatment was complicated. She recovered, but her hearing is still diminished because of the infection. I'm convinced that without her mom's insistence, Abby would not have been treated until much later in the course of her disease, and the consequences could have been disastrous.

The most important person on Abby's health care team was her mom— the only person in the universe God designed to be *her* mom. God had equipped Tonya to know her daughter in a way that no professional ever could—or should. Tonya illustrates why I believe that parents play an essential role on their child's health care team.

YOUR JOB: BEING YOUR CHILD'S HEALTH CARE QUARTERBACK

Building an effective health care team for your child is essential, and you—the parents—are the most important people on your child's health care team. To help you understand the importance of your role, let me share a football analogy I've used with my patients for years: Parents need to become their child's health care *quarterbacks*. You'll also need a good primary care physician—a medical expert who is willing to listen to you, to direct and advise you, and sometimes even to fuss at you—as your *coach*. You may need some specialists who are trained in a specific aspect of the game to be *assistant coaches*. Specialists know almost everything there is to know about a part of the body, but they can't see the entire game the same way you and your coach can. The best football teams have great quarterbacks who work with great coaches.

In the "game" that is your child's health, you, the quarterback, need to learn how to call the plays. Some parents of my patients struggled with this role. They wanted me, the doctor, to tell them what to do—to spell out which treatments or parenting techniques would be best for their children. They would indignantly tell me, "Doctor, that's *your* job, *not* mine! *Tell* me what to do." But our present health care system and culture require that parents take charge of their child's health care. You, as a parent, *must* become your child's health care quarterback.

You may be thinking, *But I'm not a medical expert, nor do I want to be. You doctors go to medical school for years to gain the expertise I desperately need when my child has a health problem. I don't want to get in your way in a crisis.*

If these are your thoughts, I understand. But there is a distinct difference between expecting (or demanding) that a physician make decisions for you and choosing a caring physician who will work in partnership with you to educate, empower, equip, enable, and expect you to participate in your child's health care responsibilities. The doctor's job is to diagnose your child's problem and make medical judgments and then to distill these into priorities and recommendations that you as a parent understand. However, the doctor may not be the best person to make most nonemergency medical decisions for your child. Your child is unique, so every medical decision is—and should be—unique. Therefore, *you* should be involved in and, ultimately, responsible for medical decisions that affect your child.

Dr. Isadore Rosenfeld, professor of clinical medicine at Cornell Medical Center, explains why you must be an active participant in your and your child's health care:

> The truth is, . . . physicians are spending less time with their patients. Many now work for insurance companies or managed care providers who have the last word on what tests or treatments they'll pay for. You may not even be told that there are better options than what you've been offered. So now, more than ever, you're essentially on your own when it comes to protecting your [child's] health and well-being.

Of course there are many ethical physicians in managed care and many caring physicians who are trying to spend more—not less—time with patients. Nevertheless, many patients and people I've spoken to on my radio and television programs tell me they feel baffled—if not powerless—in the face of the myriad of health care options. They express confusion over medical reporting in the media. As one caller told me, "One day they say TV can't hurt my child's health—and the next day they say it's harmful. Who should I believe? Can't you doctors ever get the story straight?"

The issue, I explained to the caller, is not just the doctors; to some degree, it involves the caller herself. As long as she depends completely on others—even educated professionals who may have a plethora of opinions about everything from aloe to zinc, from ADHD treatments to vaccinations—she's likely to become *more,* not less confused. A tidal wave of medical information hits us every day through morning or afternoon newspapers, national magazines, evening news shows, television magazine shows, and radio reports, plus there is a massive amount of information available on the Internet. Many times consumers hear about reports of medical studies days or even weeks before the medical journals reporting these studies arrive at doctors' offices.

It doesn't take nearly as much skill for a physician to tell you what to do as it does to educate and guide you to make your own medical decisions. Professional expertise is at its best when your child's doctor fully informs you of all the best options for your child's health care and treatment, recommends your best option in his or her professional opinion, and lets you make the final decision. When you actively participate in your child's health care in partnership with a physician who encourages and desires such teamwork, you are operating according to the best model of medicine—the one most likely to result in your child becoming highly healthy.

I always encouraged my patients, as they began to learn how to be their children's health care quarterbacks, to do at least two things: (1) Be more proactive and take more responsibility for your child's health care than you may have taken in the past, and (2) find a personal physician who will serve as your and your child's health care coach.

Dose of Wisdom

Knowledge is power. You should have as much information as possible about your condition—and your rights—so that you have the confidence to share in the decisions that affect your *health [and that of your child], the quality of* your *life, and survival itself. The better prepared you are to ask informed questions, the better your chances of receiving optimum medical care.*

Isadore Rosenfeld, M.D., health editor, Parade

For emergency medical care, of course, the model I'm proposing isn't necessary or even tenable. Certain conditions obviously require quick attention from a doctor who is well trained and experienced. A prolonged discussion of options is seldom necessary or, at times, even possible. For most of your child's medical care, however—for well-child care or chronic, potentially lifelong health problems such as attention-deficit/hyperactivity disorder (ADHD), asthma, or diabetes—it's to your advantage to learn how to be your child's health care quarterback under the guidance of a good health care coach until your child is able to take over the job.

Being your child's health care quarterback is not easy, but it is doable. For more than twenty years, this is the model I taught parents of my young patients. I'm delighted to report that the majority of parents succeeded magnificently. Sometimes they brought me cutting-edge information about treatments I hadn't yet heard about. Because of their work, I became a better doctor, and their children became healthier. So for the benefit of your child, take the time and make the effort to be your child's health care quarterback.

Resource Box   *Helpful Hints*

Navigating the Managed Care System

If you are trying to navigate the managed health care system, I recommend "Choosing and Using a Health Plan," available on the Internet from the United States Agency for Healthcare Research and Quality. You can access this website and link to the agency's consumer website through www.highlyhealthy.net.

THE PHYSICIAN'S JOB: BEING YOUR CHILD'S HEALTH CARE COACH

After you accept the job of becoming your child's health care quarterback, job number 1 is finding a suitable health care coach—your child's personal physician. Obviously, a high-quality physician is a crucial member of your child's health care team.

I highly recommend you choose a primary care physician (PCP)—such as a family physician or pediatrician—as your child's health care coach. Your child's PCP will serve as your child's generalist doctor, managing his or her overall care and working closely with you to help make most of the medical decisions you face. A PCP knows you, your child, your family, and your community, and he or she can collaborate with other health care providers, when necessary, in identifying and addressing your child's comprehensive health care needs. Having a PCP allows you to establish a trusting relationship with a doctor over time, maintain continuity in your child's health care, and move easily between crisis-oriented or acute health care problems and preventive care and health maintenance.

There is no way to accomplish the above tasks, however, if your child's doctor is unwilling or unable to take the time to provide the critical information you need and to teach you (or have his or her staff teach you) what you need to know. *But,* you may be thinking, *many times it's hard to get a doctor to stay in a room with me long enough to provide this kind of information and guidance. Most office visits seem to last less than ten minutes—and there's little I can do about it.*

To this line of reasoning, I say, "Not!" In order to get the care you want for your child, you must know that such care is available and then take steps to find it. You also must ask for this type of care and expect to receive it.

How to "Hire" a Physician to Be Your Child's Coach

Choosing the best physician to be a health care coach for your child requires gathering information. Although many insurance companies limit your choices, you should still seek a good fit. Think through and answer the following questions. The right answers can make all the difference in the world.

- Do you want a physician who is disease oriented or wellness oriented?
- Do you prefer conservative or aggressive approaches to care?
- Would you rather have a physician who is informal and warm, or formal and detached?
- Do you prefer a physician who invites your participation in your care or one who tells you what to do?
- Do you desire a male or a female physician?
- Do you prefer a physician who is interested in or at least supportive of your spiritual interests?

Once you've determined your personal preferences in a physician, ask friends, neighbors, colleagues, relatives, and clergy for doctors they'd recommend. In particular, check with people you know and trust who are connected in some way to the health care system. Always consider the opinion of other trusted providers who have cared for you or your child. If your child has specialized needs, local and state advocate or support groups can be an excellent source of information on health care providers who are skilled in these areas.

To further narrow your search, you can research the public information about prospective providers that's available through professional organizations, the Better Business Bureau, and your state's department of professional regulation and insurance. Some states also have Internet databases that allow you to investigate malpractice cases and complaints, or you may check with the clerk in the county in which the physician practices and resides. You should be able to learn if a physician is currently licensed and if the state has ever taken disciplinary action against him or her. Most states allow you to request a copy of the disciplinary order if there have been actions.

Keep in mind, however, that anyone can file a lawsuit at any time for almost any reason. The existence of a malpractice complaint or lawsuit does not automatically indicate that a physician is a bad doctor. It may mean only that a single patient was unhappy about something. Furthermore, the health outcome in question may have been out of the physician's control. However, several legal actions—or a pattern of actions—may be cause for concern.

You'll also want to consider the financial relationships between your child's doctors, your insurance company, and your hospital. If your child's doctor is hired by your employer or insurance company, the doctor may feel bound to care, first and foremost, for the needs of "the company." You want to be sure that your doctor is, first and foremost, working for your child's well-being.

Resource Box   *Helpful Hints*

The American Medical Association says it provides information on virtually every licensed physician in the United States and its possessions on its "Physician Select" website, which you can get to from www.highlyhealthy.net.

Once you've determined the doctors who are highest on your list, call their offices and ask if a staff member will take a few moments to answer your questions:

- Are you accepting new patients? Do you accept my insurance?
- How long has the doctor practiced in this area? How large is the practice?

- Does the doctor practice alone or in a group? If in a group, how many members are there and in how many offices do they practice?
- Who provides my child's care when the doctor is not available?
- At which hospitals does the doctor admit patients, and are there any limitations on the doctor's hospital privileges?
- If the doctor does not admit patients, who will care for my child if he or she has to go to the emergency room or be admitted to the hospital?
- Does a medical specialty board certify the doctor? Which board? In which specialty area?
- If I call with a question or problem, will the doctor speak to me personally—or will the nurse handle it? When is the best time to call?
- How often does the doctor recommend well-child visits and routine immunizations, and are they covered by my health plan? What does the doctor routinely check for, and which tests are generally done?
- Can a friend or family member sit in on my child's exams and procedures?
- How willing is the doctor to let me take an active role in my child's treatment? How will the doctor react if I ask about a medication or test he or she isn't familiar with or bring in my research for review?
- For an adolescent child, does the doctor insist on seeing him or her alone, or will the doctor allow me to be in the room with my child if I desire?
- How does the doctor feel about alternative medicine?

Once you choose a particular doctor, request a *brief* appointment to interview him or her. It's important to respect the physician's time. By doing so, you'll demonstrate that you are interested in a win-win doctor-patient relationship. More and more physicians who care for children are open to these interviews, which give you an opportunity to ask specific questions related to your expectations for the management of your child's health care. Increasingly, doctors offer this type of appointment at no cost. After you leave the interview, ask yourself these questions:

- Was I treated courteously and with respect? Or did I feel rushed or disrespected?
- Was the office orderly, comfortable, and clean? Did the medical facilities provide reasonable safety, comfort, and privacy?
- Was the staff friendly and helpful?
- Did I have to wait long after my appointment time to see the doctor? (You should be seen within a reasonable time for a scheduled appointment—

or be informed of any delays and given the option to see another provider or professional, reschedule your appointment, or continue waiting. A prolonged wait should occur only with your consent.)

- Were all my questions answered?
- Does the doctor emphasize *preventive* care in each of the four health wheels, as well as *acute* care?
- Do I think this doctor will provide high-quality, cost-effective, evidence-based medical treatment, regardless of my child's race, sex, religion, or national origin?

If you were not satisfied, go to the next name on your list.

Resource Box   *Helpful Hints*

The book *Examining Your Doctor* by Timothy McCall, M.D., is an excellent resource with helpful tips on how to go about finding a good doctor. It puts the white coat on you—and that horrid paper gown on your physician and hospital. You can learn more about ordering this book at my website (www.highlyhealthy.net).

Working with Your Child's Health Care Coach

If you and your child's health care coach are to work together effectively, you must communicate well. Here's a template I recommend to parents who want to work successfully with their children's doctors. This G-U-E-S-T acrostic will sharpen your skills as a health care quarterback:

G = Get the facts.
U = Understand the different layers of health care.
E = Explore treatment options.
S = Seek wise spiritual counsel.
T = Take a personal inventory.

G = Get the Facts

Whenever you face a health care decision regarding your child, ask for a thorough summary of the issue at hand. Here are some questions to consider asking your health care coach:

- What is my child's diagnosis?
- How certain are you that your diagnosis is correct?
- Which diseases or conditions other than the one being considered might this be?
- What are the possible causes of my child's condition?
- What other symptoms might be expected or are usually seen?
- Which tests or assessments are recommended for my child? What will they cost? Will they be covered by my insurance?
- Where can I learn more about this condition? What educational materials can you give me? Are there Internet sites or books you'd recommend?
- Do you know parents of other children with the same condition who are willing to share what they've learned and experienced?

If your appointment time with the doctor is too short, reschedule a longer appointment to discuss your concerns. Bring a list of all your questions, and consider bringing your spouse or a trusted friend to listen, take notes, and possibly ask questions. (This is particularly helpful if you are dealing with a serious health concern. It can be difficult to hear or remember everything a doctor says when you're under emotional stress.) If your child's doctor can't, or won't, spend the time with you that you desire, then seek one who will. This is your right and, in my opinion, your responsibility.

Double-check everything you hear and learn. If it's the truth, you'll find documentation from several sources. If the sources conflict, ask your doctor or nurse to help you sort out the contradictions. At this stage of dealing with your child's health care concerns, emphasize the gathering of useful, reliable information. It's your job to become educated about your child's condition.

U = Understand the Different Layers of Health Care

There are several levels within the health care system from which you can gain care and information.

Primary Care. For most children, the best choice for a health care coach and advocate will be a *primary care physician* (PCP), who provides the first and most basic level of medical care. These doctors are generalists (family physicians or pediatricians) trained to diagnose and treat more than 90 percent of the problems they encounter. However, there are still scores of conditions a PCP may not have the training, experience, or time to address effectively. Most are eager to help you find the kind of specialty care you need if they can't provide it. If they *can* provide the care, but you want a second or third opinion, most will gladly help you obtain these opinions.

Many PCPs have physician assistants (PAs) or nurse practitioners (NPs) in their offices. According to the Congressional Office of Technology Assessment, within their respective areas of expertise, these highly trained caregivers can provide care equivalent to that provided by physicians for the same conditions. In addition, physician assistants and nurse practitioners usually spend more time with patients than physicians—a quality many parents like.

Secondary Care. Physicians who provide secondary care are *specialists* or *subspecialists* who tend to care for a single organ system. For example, pediatric cardiologists care for problems of the heart and blood vessels in children, while pediatric neurologists care for problems of the brain, spinal cord, and nerves in children. Specialists are highly trained to care for problems in their specific areas of expertise and may be the best health care coach choice for children with certain health problems (such as sickle-cell disease, severe heart disease, and cystic fibrosis).

Tertiary Care. Children with very rare health concerns or those who require new or experimental treatments may need the care of a physician in a large medical center associated with a medical school, research center, or residency training program. These centers care for patients with the most complex medical problems. Although a PCP might see one case of a rare disease in years of practice, a medical center's physicians could treat many such cases each year.

E = Explore Treatment Options

Whenever possible, obtain complete information on the risks, benefits, and costs of each suggested treatment option. Always ask each health care expert you consult, "What are *all* the potential treatments available, and how do you suggest we analyze them in order to come up with the best treatment for my child?"

Ask how your child's condition can be expected to progress with or without treatment. Even for the most commonly recommended options, ask your physician, "Will you discuss with me all of the possible risks and benefits of what you are recommending? What will this cost? Of these costs, how much will I need to pay?"

Sadly, many doctors aren't used to caring for children of parents who are health care quarterbacks and may seem annoyed by these types of discussions.

If your child's doctor seems bothered or rushed, consider saying, "Doctor, you seem rushed [or busy or bothered]. Would there be a better time to discuss these concerns?"

When a friend of mine asked her doctor a question like this, she was told, "I'm not sure I'll *ever* have the time for this type of thing."

"No problem," she calmly replied. "Can you suggest another doctor who does?"

Her child's doctor smiled. He got the point. From then on, he made time for her. If he hadn't, she was prepared to go elsewhere to obtain the assistance she needed.

S = Seek Wise Spiritual Counsel

Spiritual counsel is a critical component of your child's health care, especially if your child faces a life-threatening situation. If your faith community has staff pastors or elders, make an appointment with them to inform them of your child's condition and ask for their prayers, advice, and support. Pastors and elders are usually comfortable helping parents whose children face health-related situations. They may ask you challenging questions about your or your child's spiritual health and are often able to give you wise counsel. They may also put you in touch with people in the congregation or local community who have wrestled with similar health conditions.

If your faith community doesn't have staff pastors or elders, schedule a visit with a pastoral professional you trust. If you aren't involved in a faith community, ask your friends to recommend a pastoral professional—most of whom are well trained and willing to counsel parents who are wrestling with health care decisions. Or consider calling your local hospital's chaplain. Most hospitals have chaplains who would be delighted to assist you as you seek wisdom and comfort during a medical dilemma or crisis.

T = Take a Personal Inventory

Begin a personal inventory—in writing—of your child's health care needs. Buy a notebook specifically for this purpose, and set aside quiet time each day to think, meditate, pray, and journal. Don't just record facts. Record what trusted family members and friends say about your child's condition and the treatments you're considering. Record how you feel about your child's medical, emotional, relational, and spiritual challenges, as well as the ones you're facing. Write honestly. This journal is for your eyes only.

As part of your inventory, carefully consider what your intuition is telling you about your child's medical problems. If you weren't afraid of any consequences, what would you do? If money were no object, what would you do? What do you feel God is leading you to do or not do?

You may also choose to write out your prayers and record any answers. Spend plenty of time listening to answers that will come to you through your spiritual ears, the wise guidance of others, and the circumstances that unfold.

Finally, write about the support you and your child need now and during the course of treatment. What support is available to you? Where might you find additional support?

Making Well-Informed Decisions

Following the G-U-E-S-T steps can help you make fully informed, educated, spiritually sound, and wise health care decisions for your child. But I hasten to add a caveat here. Some of my patients believed that following the G-U-E-S-T process would *guarantee* good results. It will not. It can only improve your child's chances for the best possible outcomes.

Resource Box   *Helpful Hints*

Concerned about Preventing Medical Errors?

An article containing suggestions for preventing medical errors can be found on my website: www.highlyhealthy.net.

Being informed about your child's options, expected outcomes, and possible complications or side effects beforehand dramatically reduces the potential for anger or disappointment should a less than desirable outcome occur. Most disappointment or anger results from unmet expectations—disappointment if the expectation is lightly held, anger if the expectation is strongly held. For example, you expect a certain outcome for your child, whether it was spelled out by your physician or just implied. Complications you weren't warned about arise. Side effects you didn't know about before you started giving your child a certain medication surface. These kinds of unexpected outcomes result in disappointment or anger—emotions that are not highly healthy.

In contrast, when you become your child's health care quarterback, you ask questions *before* treatment is started. You compare the benefits of the prescribed treatment with the complications or side effects it might create. You become aware—in advance—of the chances for your child's full recovery and tend to experience fewer surprises.

But there is no way in this imperfect world, even when you take full personal responsibility for your child's health care and work with the doctor to prevent problems, that you can ever completely control the outcome. If you and your child have a healthy spiritual wheel, however, you can be assured that Someone is controlling the outcome. According to Romans 8:28 in the Bible, God works in *all* things (good and bad) for the good of those who have a personal relationship with him, love him, and live according to his plan and purposes. Even though we cannot be perfect health care quarterbacks, we can all choose to know and trust the One who is.

Resource Box   **Helpful Hints**

What If My Doctor and I Don't See Eye to Eye about My Child's Care?

If you don't understand or agree with the course of treatment your child's doctor recommends, don't panic. It's not so unusual. Here are some things you can do:

1. Don't be afraid to ask the doctor (or nurse) specific questions. Make sure you understand the doctor's recommendations and the reasons behind them. Always ask about alternative treatments. If you forget to ask a question, call when you get home or discuss it during your next visit.
2. Seek a second opinion. It never hurts to get more than one opinion, especially if your child's problem is not routine. It's your right to have the information you need to make a wise decision. If your child's doctor is uncomfortable with getting a second opinion, I think you should be uncomfortable with your child's doctor. Health insurance plans usually pay for a second opinion.
3. You have a right to change doctors if you consistently find yourself at odds with your child's physician.
4. If you ever suspect that your child's doctor has withheld proper medical care or provided inappropriate care, discuss it with the

doctor or one of the doctor's staff members. If you are not satisfied, call your health plan. Ask to speak with a patient advocate whose job it is to help you resolve such problems. Most health plans have a medical director or a board of doctors who don't belong to the plan who can discuss your situation with you and objectively review your case. If you remain unsatisfied, contact your employer's representative, who may be able to help you resolve the problem or help you decide whether to file a grievance. You can contact your state department of insurance or the state medical society to file a grievance.

Dose of Wisdom

Practice an attitude of gratitude with your child's physician. If you already have a winning health care team and don't need new players, write a brief thank-you note to your child's health care providers. Many of them hear only complaints. Rare is the appreciative patient who will write just to say, "You're doing a great job caring for my child, and I appreciate you so much."

Dr. Walt Larimore

OTHER PLAYERS ON YOUR CHILD'S HEALTH CARE TEAM

Diane was a first-time mom. Her fifteen-month-old son, Tommy, seemed perfect. Yet, Diane's mom thought Tommy wasn't quite right. This grandmother thought his language was developing slowly. He seemed to communicate more with gestures than words, to prefer to be left alone, to be overly sensitive to touch, and to be agitated or cry when held. Nevertheless, Diane wasn't concerned; as his physician, neither was I. The grandmother, however, was concerned enough to attend Tommy's fifteen-month well-child visit to express her observations. I tried to reassure her, but she insisted that Tommy be evaluated at a nearby developmental center.

I was always delighted when my patients sought second opinions. Virtually every time I learned more, and so did the parents of my young patients.

In this case, I was shocked when the developmental center concluded that Tommy had one of the autistic variant disorders! Both Diane and I would have realized that something was wrong as Tommy got older, but we had missed the subtle, early signs of autism. The grandmother was right on target—and because of the grandmother's intuition and sharp observation, Tommy was able to enter treatment far earlier than most children (the earlier the treatment for autistic disorders starts, the better the results).

Family and Friends

Most parents of the children I cared for as a family physician did not consider the possibility that their extended family and friends could or should be part of their health care team. Yet, as was true in Tommy's case, these individuals can play a crucial role. Studies show that family and friends are consistently rated as a vital support for parents whose children are going through major health crises. They can also be a great source of advice on parenting. Yet, as helpful as most family members and friends can be, the potential is there for some of them to harm your child or introduce values that you consider harmful and unhealthy. Thus, you need to be able to fire family members or friends who negatively affect your children's health.

But, you may ask, *what if I have no family in town?* or *What if I'm a single parent?* or *What if I've just moved to a new town and have no friends?* If one of these describes your situation, you need to begin recruiting additional members for your child's health care team. I'm convinced that your child's health depends on it.

I think of Margie, who was shocked when her husband of fifteen years moved out without warning to live with a young woman he met on the Internet. He left her with three boys, ages seven, nine, and twelve, and no financial support. Margie had to quickly find a job to support her family. Overnight her boys became latchkey children, and it wasn't long before they began to get into trouble. Margie consulted me about her symptoms of insomnia, anxiety, and depression.

As we talked, I realized that Margie needed help and needed it fast. She had too few members on her team. She didn't need a prescription for a sleeping pill, anti-anxiety pill, or antidepressant; she needed to build a support team.

With Margie's permission, I called her pastor, and he quickly contacted a group of single moms in the church, who eagerly included Margie in their support group. The pastor recruited a small group of men in the church who agreed to assist Margie with running errands, doing chores, and—most important—

mentoring her boys. With Margie's support, I called the psychologist at the boys' schools and arranged for male mentors to assist them at school. I also encouraged Margie to recruit help from her extended family. They did not live near her, but they leaped into action when she suggested specific ways they could help.

Although Margie's situation remained difficult, things improved when she built and utilized a small network of friends and family to help her and her children become more highly healthy. What could have become a lonely, isolated, angry, and bitter single mom with kids spinning out of control became a much healthier family unit.

Dr. J. W. Pennebaker, author of *Opening Up: The Healing Power of Confiding in Others,* concurs that having family members and friends on your—and your child's—health care team is critical to your health and that of your child, especially to the extent that you feel comfortable expressing your emotions about your trials and tribulations. It's not just having family members and friends, though; it's sharing, confessing, and being vulnerable within those relationships that helps protect and improve your health, which in turn has a positive impact on your child's health. Dr. Pennebaker explains: "Here's the kicker. If you have had a trauma that you have not talked about with anyone, the number of friends you have is unrelated to your health. Social support only protects your health if you use it wisely . . . merely having friends is not enough." Having close relationships with at least a small number of friends or family members is essential to creating a winning health care team.

Resource Box   **Helpful Hints**

Connecting in Community

The Bible teaches that human beings are not designed to be loners. We are meant to be part of a community—what the Bible calls a living "body." Ideally, this body is like a family to us. When Jesus prayed for those who would become his followers, he prayed that they would support and care for each other in unity and harmony. Read the following Bible verses for more on connecting in community: Genesis 2:18; Acts 2:42; 1 Corinthians 12:12–27; 2 Corinthians 6:14–18; John 17:11, 21–22.

Support Groups

If your child is dealing with a chronic health issue, or if you're facing tough parenting issues in general, you'll also benefit from including another group of players on your health care team—those who wrestle with health issues that are the same as or similar to the ones you and your child face. In addition to providing a great forum for the dissemination of useful information and the sharing of personal experiences, these groups help prevent or alleviate isolation, alienation, and loneliness. They demonstrate the healing power of sharing and listening. Although the people in these groups usually start out as strangers, this kind of anonymous setting makes it easier for some people to open up and be vulnerable.

Support groups take a variety of forms. Some focus on a particular disease process such as ADHD, learning disorders, diabetes, autism, or asthma. Others focus on parenting skills or the issues faced by single parents. Still others focus on emotional issues such as depression, anxiety, and bipolar disease. You can locate such groups through local hospitals, national associations, faith communities, physicians, and mental health professionals.

You may find dozens of Internet support groups that deal with health issues and decisions that are the same as or similar to those you and your child face. These may be helpful to you, but a couple of warnings are in order: (1) An Internet support group can never provide the level of personal support and healing potential provided by a group of people with whom you meet face-to-face, and (2) much of the medical advice provided through Internet chat rooms, bulletin boards, or support group websites is inaccurate and sometimes dangerous.

Mentors

If there is a lost art in America, it is the art of mentoring. The Bible encourages older and wiser men and women to guide the younger and less experienced —yet many in this category fail in this regard. I'm thankful for Bill and Jane Judge, the mentors on whom Barb and I depended. Bill and I met almost every Tuesday for nearly sixteen years. He would guide me, listen to me, pray for me, and counsel, advise, teach, correct, and admonish me. As couples, we often double-dated, and the two of them would counsel us and answer our questions. During those years, Barb and I faced scores of health decisions related to our children and ourselves. Bill and Jane's mentoring helped us become a healthier family.

Faith Community Members and Bible Study and Prayer Partners

Socialization has a positive effect on health, and socialization in a faith community is exceptionally good for your and your child's health. As you deal with your child's health, it's important for you and your child to have people who will pray with you and for you and your child. *But I'm not into praying,* you may be thinking. Then you should know that prayer affects a wide variety of health outcomes, including such issues as anxiety, depression, disabilities, marital satisfaction, pain, and generalized well-being. In addition, researchers have demonstrated that the "strongest factors for well-being (life-satisfaction and happiness) were frequency of prayer and prayer experience."

Prayer has been deemed so important that some hospitals now ask parents if they desire prayer before and during surgery—for them and their child. If they do, the hospital staff calls a local group that is devoted to prayer to provide this important health care service. A physician friend who is the head of a pediatric intensive care unit at a large city hospital has worked with the chaplains on his hospital's staff so that all patients who consent are prayed for every day of their hospital stay.

Mental Health Professionals

You may be surprised that I've included this section, but children are experiencing mental health disorders in epidemic numbers. In the United States, health professionals are seeing soaring rates of ADHD, anxiety, depression, learning disorders, and bipolar disease in children and adolescents. According to the National Mental Health Association, one in five children has a diagnosable mental, emotional, learning, eating, or behavioral disorder. And up to one in ten may suffer from a serious emotional disturbance. As many as one in every thirty-three children and one in eight adolescents may be clinically depressed. Yet 70 percent of these children do not receive mental health services.

Psychologists, professional counselors, and social workers are licensed, certified, and trained to provide diagnosis and therapy for a variety of mental, emotional, and relational problems in children. In most states they do not prescribe medication and often work in conjunction with primary care physicians. Pastoral counselors and chaplains can be of great help with spiritual problems, as well as with certain emotional and relational problems, but if your child faces more severe emotional or relational issues I'd usually recommend seeing a licensed therapist in one of the mental health disciplines.

Child psychiatrists—medical doctors who are specially trained in evaluating and treating mental health and disease in children—also play an important role on the health care teams for some children. Unlike other mental health professionals, they can prescribe medications, order laboratory and other diagnostic tests, and admit patients to the hospital. Very often child psychiatrists work with a team of mental health professionals.

Resource Box   *Helpful Hints*

To find a faith-based counselor in your area, call the counseling department at Focus on the Family (1-800-A-FAMILY). Patients who desire faith-based counseling can call the Meier Clinics (1-800-7-CLINIC), New Life Clinics (1-800-NEW-LIFE), or the Rapha Counseling Clinics (1-800-383-HOPE). You can access my website (www.highlyhealthy.net) to learn more about these resources.

Registered Dietitians

You may—or may not—realize that the average physician who cares for children has little or no training in nutrition. Yet, as I'll discuss in the next chapter, nutritional habits can significantly affect your child's physical, emotional, and relational health wheels. Today there is an epidemic of overweight and obese children and adolescents in the United States. Registered dietitians, who are well trained in nutrition and the dietary management of many health conditions, are providing invaluable advice to physicians, parents, and children. Many registered dietitians have private practices; others serve on the staff of local hospitals and are available for private consultation. All are licensed by their respective states.

If your family's nutritional habits need repair, ask your child's doctor to refer you to a dietitian for a consultation. He or she will take a careful diet history and suggest strategies for improving your family's nutritional health. It may be one of the best consultations you'll ever experience, as was the case for the Roflinger family.

I had the privilege of caring for Bill, Sherry, and their four children. The entire family was overweight and experiencing health difficulties. They consistently resisted my suggestion to take charge and make nutrition-related changes—until Bill's dad dropped dead of a heart attack at the age of fifty-eight. Then they became *very* interested.

Our local hospital dietitians offered a nutrition class for community residents each week. I suggested that the entire family commit to attending these classes for three months. They did. They learned to cook their favorite meals in healthier ways. They learned how to dine together and how doing so would benefit their family life. They learned about portion control, good versus bad sugars, and good versus bad fats. They even learned how to exercise as a family.

I wish you could've seen them one year later! They were all approaching their ideal body weight. Bill was off blood pressure medication, and Sherry was off diabetic medication. The children looked and felt good. The entire family had received positive feedback from friends. They were well along the road to becoming healthy!

Pharmacists

Along with your child's primary care physician, your child's pharmacist may be one of the most important members of your child's health care team. Pharmacists can guide parents in the appropriate use of both prescription and nonprescription medications, as well as over-the-counter products, herbs, vitamins, and supplements. They can also give direction to parents in avoiding overdoses and interactions from these agents.

Clergy or Pastoral Professionals

A spiritual adviser is a wise addition to your health care team. Pastors, priests, rabbis, and other spiritual professionals such as chaplains and pastoral counselors are obvious selections. In many faith communities, elders, deacons, or specially trained lay leaders also provide spiritual guidance for parents. Of course, youth pastors may be one of *the* most valuable additions to your child's health care team.

Resource Box **Helpful Hints**

Take a Spiritual Inventory

Finding a doctor and other health care team members who share your spiritual foundation and practice is fairly simple if you use a spiritual inventory. Increasingly doctors use spiritual inventories (or histories) in their care of patients. Just as a doctor can inquire about a patient's spiritual beliefs, a parent can ask about a doctor's beliefs and practices related to medical care. Health care givers may be surprised to be asked the questions in the spiritual inventory—I suspect it rarely happens—but they should be perfectly willing to let you know where they stand on these issues.

Here's something to remember: Because the process of finding players for your health care team applies to alternative or complementary caregivers as well as physicians, it can be crucial to ask these questions. Why? Because at least some alternative practitioners use their therapy to recruit unsuspecting patients into spiritual belief systems I consider to be highly unhealthy.

Consider asking the following questions during your interview or during your first official appointment with your health care provider. I realize that most parents wouldn't ask all of these questions, especially during a first meeting. However, if your spirituality is very important to you and you desire a health care provider who shares your beliefs, it may be useful eventually to discuss these questions. (I have no doubt that you'll have your own questions to add to this list.)

- Are you willing to consider my religious or spiritual preferences as you care for my child?
- Are you open to discussing the religious or spiritual implications of my child's health care?
- Are you willing to work with my spiritual mentors (such as pastor, priest, rabbi, elder) and other members of my health care team (family, friends, mentor, support group, and so on) in providing my child with the best possible health care?
- Are you willing to pray with me, or for my child, if we feel we need prayer?
- What does spirituality mean to you? How much is your religious faith a source of strength and comfort to you?

PLAYERS YOU MAY NOT WANT TO INCLUDE ON YOUR CHILD'S HEALTH CARE TEAM

Chiropractors

A chiropractor is a health care provider who utilizes musculoskeletal therapies such as manipulation, stretching, and other physical therapies. You need to be aware that, through the years, chiropractic care has separated into two camps: *traditional chiropractors,* who adhere strictly to the original philosophy of locating and eliminating what they call "subluxations" (misalignments of the spine), and *holistic chiropractors,* who combine musculoskeletal manipulation and adjustments with other therapies such as gentle stretching, trigger-point treatments, hot or cold treatments, nutrition counseling and therapies, supplement recommendations, and exercise programs.

During my years of practice in Central Florida, some of my adolescent and adult patients and I did benefit from the services of a holistic, science-based chiropractor committed to playing a part in a traditional health care team. The patients who most benefited from this type of chiropractic care had acute musculoskeletal injuries, especially some forms of neck and back pain. However, I never used chiropractic services for young children. In fact, most child care experts believe that chiropractors have virtually no place on a child's health care team.

Be alert for the following danger signs:

- *Subluxation theory.* Many chiropractors believe that disease is caused by misalignments of the spine—what they call *subluxations*—that pinch nerves going from the spinal column to other parts of the body. They believe that after proper manipulation or adjustment, normal nerve transmissions are restored and the body resumes its innate ability to recover from, or even prevent, illness. From my viewpoint, and the viewpoint of the overwhelming majority of doctors and researchers, there is virtually no scientific evidence for this theory.
- *Recruitment practices.* Parents must be aware that some practice-building programs for chiropractors are based on pediatric care. I caution you about chiropractors who try to recruit mothers-to-be and children into receiving expensive, unnecessary, and potentially dangerous care.
- *Immunization misinformation.* Another major problem concerning chiropractic care for children is that many chiropractors have unscientific views about the risks and value of immunizations. A significant number of chiropractors in the United States do not promote vaccinations.

Because of these concerns, I join many child care experts, primary care physicians, and researchers who would agree with Samuel Homola, a practicing chiropractor for forty-three years, in his assessment of chiropractic care for children: "Chiropractors do not have adequate training in the diagnosis and treatment of pediatric ailments. And they do not have recourse to antibiotics and other medical treatment methods that are essential in combating potentially fatal or crippling illnesses."

A related discussion of the issues surrounding the use of chiropractic care with children can be found in appendix 3 (pages 299–300).

Other Alternative Health Care Providers

The growing interest in alternative medicine among adults has carried over to children and into the offices of pediatricians and family practitioners. Parents wonder if echinacea, a popular but scientifically unproven remedy for preventing colds, should be given to a child with a runny nose. Is garlic oil a better eardrop than commercial products made specifically for children? What about acupuncture for children with cerebral palsy, or megavitamin, herbal, or supplement therapy for children with ADHD? A survey by the American Academy of Pediatrics found that 93 percent of pediatrician members reported being asked about alternative therapies by parents of their patients. Another survey found that 2 percent of parents in the United States use alternative medicine with their children.

Parents use alternative therapies and herbal remedies for their children for the same reasons they use them on themselves: They believe they are cheaper or safer. However, nothing could be further from the truth than the belief that if something is natural, it must be safe. The reason herbal remedies work, when they do, is because they *do* alter the body's chemistry. Many parents forget that most alternative practitioners, particularly those who deal in nutritional therapy, are unlicensed and unregulated. Furthermore, such therapies are, with rare exception, not tested, proven, or approved for use in children. All natural therapies have potential adverse reactions, and most can react with at least some over-the-counter or prescription medications.

Resource Box   Helpful Hints

In *Alternative Medicine: The Christian Handbook,* you can read about what Dónal O'Mathúna and I discovered as we researched the most popular alternative therapies, herbal remedies, vitamins, and dietary supplements available in today's health marketplace. We looked at the evidence to support each therapy for each disease or condition it was supposed to treat and considered underlying spiritual issues that might affect a patient's decision to use or avoid a particular therapy. To find out more about this book, go to www.highlyhealthy.net.

Parents who wish to find out more about particular herbs, vitamins, and supplements have free access to the world's largest and most trustworthy database on herbs, vitamins, and supplements (The Natural Medicines Comprehensive Database) through my website at www.highlyhealthy.net.

It will be many years before a broad range of therapies and herbal remedies can be adequately tested to ensure the safety and effectiveness of their use with children. Until then, parents might limit their exploration of alternative treatments to those that do not alter the body's chemistry, such as acupuncture and acupressure. Children should never be given herbal remedies or megadoses of vitamins in the belief that they are safer than pharmaceuticals. We still know too little about what works and what doesn't, about the appropriate preparation and the proper dosage for age and body weight, to be able to safely use such potentially dangerous products for children. Until studies show that a particular alternative therapy is safe and effective for children, that therapy should be avoided. The potential risks are too high. Also, parents who are considering treating their children with alternative therapies should also keep in mind that many alternative medicine practitioners have little conventional medical training.

If you choose to add alternative, complementary, or herbal therapies to your child's health care, or if you seek the services of an alternative practitioner for your child, be sure to do so under the direction and supervision of your health care coach—your child's primary care physician.

A related discussion of the issues surrounding the use of alternative care with children can be found in appendix 3 (pages 301–2).

If you're like most parents, I bet you hadn't thought about becoming your child's health care quarterback. I hope you see how valuable and essential your role as quarterback is. The steps I've outlined will help ensure that you are building the best health care team for your child. It takes work on your part, but no person on earth is better qualified or prepared for the job.

Medical studies show that adults who actively participate in their own medical care (who are their own health care quarterbacks) are not only more likely to receive better medical care but are less likely to experience medical errors and mistakes. My belief is that the same will be proven in the health care of children. This is clearly one of the foundational principles for your children as they walk the path to becoming highly healthy.

Chapter Five

Ensure Proper Nutrition

B arb and I were approaching middle age and our children were approaching adolescence when we all realized our readings on the bathroom scales were higher than we cared to admit. One night we sat down to discuss the issue. We knew we weren't exercising enough, that we ate out at fast-food restaurants more than we should, and that our diets were higher in sugar and saturated fat than was healthy. We had also gotten away from eating together as a family and were eating some meals in front of the television. We knew we needed to improve, but instead of making changes, we decided to keep a daily diary of what we ate.

At the end of one month, we had another family discussion. We discovered we had eaten only nine dinners together as a family. All of us had avoided breakfast and had consumed a surprising number of soft drinks and an unexpected amount of snack food. Our meeting ended with a decision to do some fact-finding.

Barb and I viewed our parenting role as one in which we were continually reading about and learning how to be better parents. If we wanted to improve our children's nutrition, we needed some education—and we needed to improve our own nutritional habits. During the next two weeks, we read books on improving our family's nutrition. We learned the difference between good and bad fats, carbohydrates and proteins. We learned about our children's varying nutritional needs. We learned how to select snacks low in "bad" saturated fats or trans fats and "bad" sugars. All this reading, along with my medical training and a review of pertinent medical studies, convinced us that nutrition and exercise were essential to our health and our children's health.

Nutritional habits are not as easily taught as they are caught. Barb and I came to the sober realization that we needed to demonstrate good nutrition before our children would practice good nutrition. We came to understand the necessity of good exercise and activity habits for our children, which meant we needed to do those activities right along with them.

Armed with facts and ideas, we were prepared to make some key decisions at our next family meeting—decisions that have positively influenced our family's health ever since. We changed our nutrition and exercise habits. As a result, we feel better, have more energy, sleep better, and have lost weight.

Barb and I just wish we had made these changes when our children were younger—and we're not alone in this desire. A national survey of parents indicated that almost 70 percent want their children to have good nutrition and eating habits. However, only 40 percent said they've succeeded in this area of parenting. Why this discrepancy between desire and success? Most parents aren't willing to practice what they preach. Only 51 percent of parents rate exercising and being physically fit as absolutely essential to impress on their children. In addition, more than nine out of every ten parents say they let their child eat junk food. And 20 percent of parents let their children eat junk food constantly.

The startling statistics in this national survey pinpointed what I saw in my practice and in my own family: We parents are failing to teach good eating habits, and it's not because we lack information and knowledge. If we want our children to be highly healthy, we must model good nutrition and eating habits. Furthermore, it's *much* easier to teach these principles to children when they are young than to wait, as we did, until their teenage years.

A 2003 national survey of over three thousand infants and toddlers showed that very young American children (four months to twenty-four months of age) are being fed poorly—with too much fat, sugar, and salt and too few fruits and vegetables. One-third of these children were fed no fruits or vegetables—and for those who were, fries were the most common selection.

There's no better time than before age five to make a lifelong impact on your child's nutritional habits—an impact that will contribute to disease prevention for years to come. If we do not model healthy nutritional habits, our children may suffer grave consequences.

THE TERRIBLE DANGERS OF CHILDHOOD OBESITY

I was with Sarah when she took her last breath. She didn't die from a car accident, a drowning, or a gunshot wound. She died from obesity.

I first saw Sarah for her three-year-old well-child visit. She was already overweight. Her baby bottle was filled with a soft drink. Through the years I cajoled, coaxed, pleaded with, beseeched, implored, encouraged, and appealed to her parents and family to change their ways. They did not.

Sarah's first hospitalization for diabetes occurred when she was only eight years old. High blood pressure began at age ten. Her family's lack of attention to these problems led to asthma, heart problems, and scores of hospitalizations. Finally, at age fourteen, Sarah's body gave out. Her last admission was for a diabetic coma that led to a massive heart attack and death. When she died, I cried.

Being overweight or obese is a serious threat to a child's health. Childhood obesity—and the physical, emotional, relational, and spiritual diseases it brings—is now epidemic. Although Sarah's case is extreme, as many as one in three children in the United States today may be overweight or obese! In 1970, only about 4 percent of six- to eleven-year-olds were obese. By 2000, the rate had increased to more than 15 percent.

Being overweight or obese during childhood or adolescence dramatically increases the risk of obesity during adulthood. This increased risk is due to poor eating or exercise habits developed during childhood, metabolic and hormonal changes caused by being overweight or obese, and eating abnormalities based on the poor self-esteem and depression often associated with obesity. Childhood obesity also increases the risk of childhood diseases that were rare when I entered medicine in the 1970s. Such diseases include type 2 diabetes, high blood pressure, early hardening of the arteries, soaring cholesterol levels, sleep apnea, stomach and pancreas disease, liver and gall bladder disease, increased cardiovascular risk factors, early arthritis, and many more. In fact, the American Heart Association estimates that 27 million American children under the age of nineteen have high cholesterol and that 2.2 million have high blood pressure. Type 2 diabetes is considered epidemic in adolescents. In fact, the U.S. Centers for Disease Control and Prevention (CDC) predicts that one in three American children born in 2000 will go on to develop diabetes. And up to 50 percent of children with these diseases don't even know they have them!

Childhood obesity can yield emotional and social trauma as well. For years we've known that chubby children are teased and bullied by their classmates, which can lead to low self-esteem. Not until recently did we learn how badly obesity affects children emotionally and socially. In 2003, University of California researchers compared quality of life scores of obese children with those of healthy, normal-weight children and children with cancer who have had chemotherapy. Obese children were five and one-half times as likely to report an impaired quality of life as healthy, normal-weight children. Even more shocking, severely obese children rate their quality of life as about the same as children with cancer who have been treated with chemotherapy!

In addition, children or teens who are obese or overweight are often considered to be lazy when, in reality, physical activity is much more difficult for them than for children of normal weight. Excessive weight stresses children's joints and may cause leg or back pain when they exercise. Obesity also reduces their endurance, making exercise more difficult. Last, but not least, low self-esteem or depression, which often accompanies being overweight or obese, alters the production of brain chemicals that influence the desire for activity.

Children or teens who become obese will have significantly more difficulty losing weight and maintaining weight loss throughout life. Why is this? Because children or teens who become overweight or obese do so by dramatically increasing the number *and* the size of their fat cells. Obese children may have five times more fat cells than leaner children. *Why is this so bad?* you may be thinking. *Can't you lose them later, when you lose weight?*

No! Emphatically, no! Weight loss will cause a decrease in fat cell size but *not* fat cell numbers. Therefore, a critical part of raising highly healthy children is preventing them from becoming overweight or obese.

FACING THE THREATS TO YOUR CHILD'S NUTRITIONAL HEALTH

What can you do to diminish this terrible threat to your children's health and overall well-being? Don't give up. You *can* make positive changes, and the earlier you start, the better.

Innumerable studies show that childhood eating and exercise habits are more easily changed than adult habits, but we parents must be willing to make these changes, too. We must resist the temptation to rationalize and say that obesity "runs in the family." The fact that obesity has become epidemic during the last three decades suggests that environmental and behavioral factors have played the most significant roles. So let's explore some positive steps you can take to help your children become more highly healthy.

Turn Off the Television and Get Some Exercise

The CDC believes that a reduction in physical activity is the major cause of childhood obesity. Simply put, a person becomes overweight or obese when the calories taken in exceed the calories burned. An increase in calorie intake or a decrease in calories utilized (a decrease in physical activity) will produce fat accumulation and weight gain. Recent studies have demonstrated that television and computer use by children is one cause of reduced physical activity.

Children are watching significantly more television now than in the past. One study showed that children who watch five or more hours of television per day are five times more likely to be overweight or obese than those who watch less than two hours per day. Instead of playing outside—running, riding a bike, playing ball—children who watch television are more sedentary, allowing more calories to be converted to fat.

Television contributes to obesity in other ways as well:

- Watching television significantly reduces the metabolic rate—the rate at which the body burns calories.
- Slick commercials, especially those shown during programming aimed at children, actively encourage viewers to buy and eat foods containing high amounts of saturated ("bad") fat and simple ("bad") sugars. One study showed that 80 percent of all advertisements aired during children's programs promote unhealthy foods!
- When children (or adults, for that matter) snack or eat meals in front of the television, they subconsciously teach themselves to feel hungry in front of the television—whether or not they are, in fact, hungry.

Decreasing the number of hours a child watches television will typically reduce the number of snacks consumed, increase activity levels, and cause a significant loss in body weight. So as often as possible, Barb and I turned off the television and computer and took our children outside to play. Increased physical activity allowed them to burn calories before they became fat. It boosted their energy expenditure and sped up their metabolism so they could better use the calories they took in. With more exercise, they slept better, performed better in school, and behaved better.

Even with no change in your child's body weight or fatness, exercise has multiple health benefits. One study has shown that fifty minutes of exercise just three times per week improves blood cholesterol levels (and other lipids) and blood pressure. However, exercise alone does not make children highly healthy. It is most effective when coupled with better nutrition and eating habits.

Dose of Wisdom

Although encouraging our children to be outside worked well, getting out and exercising with them was even better! Increase your quantity *time and your* quality *time with your children by playing together, riding bicycles together, taking nature walks in the park, and so on.*

Dr. Walt Larimore

Limit or Eliminate the Fast Food

Many years ago, Barb and I pulled off the highway to get gas and eat lunch at a fast-food diner. I ordered a broiled chicken breast with potatoes, gravy, and a biscuit, which I thought was a healthy lunch. I should have known better when I had to excuse myself to wash my greasy fingers. On the way back to the table, I passed a nutritional chart and looked up my meal. My "healthy" meal had 920 calories and more than 50 grams of fat! I was shocked, but I shouldn't have been.

Every day significant numbers of Americans eat at fast-food restaurants. The food is inexpensive, tasty, and convenient. But—and this is a big *but*—fast food is usually loaded with saturated fat and calories and is extremely low in fiber and nutrients. Just so you know how bad fast food really is, consider the following sampling:

As of this writing, a Big N' Tasty with large fries and a Diet Coke has 1,080 calories, 58 grams of fat, and 14.5 grams of saturated fat. Add cheese, and you add 50 calories, 5 grams of fat, and 2 grams of saturated fat. Yet an average adult needs only about 2,000 calories each day, and *no* saturated, or "bad," fat!

At another of my favorite fast-food restaurants, I would order an Extra-Long Cheese Coney with large Tater Tots and a medium Vanilla Coke. The chili-and-cheese dog by itself has 666 calories, 42 grams of fat, and 17 grams of saturated fat. The potatoes and the soda add 596 calories, 21 fat grams, and 4 saturated fat grams.

Six Krispy Kreme doughnut holes provide 440 calories, with more than 50 percent (220) of those calories from fat (13 grams of total fat, 3 grams of saturated fat).

If your child orders a Big Mac with a super-size fries and a large soda, he or she gets 1,500 calories, about 40 percent of those from fat. For a small child, that's a day or a day and a half's worth of calories!

The impact of fast-food restaurants on the nation's culture, economy, and diet is hard to overstate. Almost every American child eats at a McDonald's at least once a month. In his revealing book *Fast Food Nation,* author Eric Schlosser points to a survey of American schoolchildren that found that 96 percent could identify Ronald McDonald. The only fictional character with a higher degree of recognition was Santa Claus! Last year, the typical American ate about thirty pounds of fries, mostly at fast-food restaurants, making fries the most-ordered dish at American restaurants. According to Schlosser, we parents spend more money on fast food for our families than we do on higher education, personal computers, software, or new cars. And, he says, we spend more on fast food than on movies, books, magazines, newspapers, videos, and recorded music combined!

I'll explain more about making healthier food choices later in this chapter. Right now, simply recognize that reducing your family's visits to fast-food restaurants and eating fewer fast-food snacks and home-delivered fast foods (such as pizza) can be a highly healthy step.

Eat Together as a Family

Most of us think more about what our children are eating than how and where they're eating it. Yet, how and where make a big difference. Experts tell us that making family meals a priority is more than worth the effort.

A study published in the American Psychological Association newsletter found that teenagers who ate with their families five times or more a week were less likely to do drugs or be depressed, were more motivated at school, and had better peer relationships. A survey of National Merit Scholars from the past twenty years found that, without exception, these amazing students came from families who ate together three or more nights a week. Not only are family meals associated with smarter children; spending quality meal time together contributes to their emotional and spiritual growth. It's when you're together, sharing the details of your day, that real bonding happens.

Barb and I considered it extremely important for our family to sit together at the table for breakfast *and* supper as often as possible. When we ate together as a family, we could enjoy being a family. It was a time to find out what everyone was going to do, or had done, that day. It was also a time for Barb and me to share our values with Kate and Scott. Of course, it wasn't always easy to accomplish this. We aimed for five dinners a week, but because of our varied schedules it was sometimes only one or two dinners a week. By starting our family dining routine when our children were young, it was easier to stick to it as they grew older and busier. As they matured, Kate and Scott looked forward to our family mealtimes as much as we did.

Barb, who was trained as a teacher, believes that family meals provide an opportunity to boost social and language skills, even for babies. She believes that the more words children hear, the more stimulation they receive and the more readily they will want to be part of the family. I must admit, her theory seems like a good one to me.

Great family meals don't just happen by accident. They are the result of deliberate decisions and actions. The following tried-and-true guidelines from the Larimore home may help you create mealtimes that everyone will cherish.

- *Prepare the meal together.* When Kate and Scott helped Barb prepare a meal, they received real-life lessons in nutrition and hands-on math practice (as they helped measure or count ingredients). Barb also realized that children who have been involved in the cooking process are more likely to eat the results!
- *Leave the television off during meals.* Eating in front of the television makes it extremely difficult to pay attention to feelings of fullness and can lead to overeating. What's more, when you're watching television, you're not interacting as a family.
- *Refuse to answer phone calls during meals.* If you have an answering machine or voice mail system, use it during mealtimes.
- *Resist the urge to fuss or lecture during mealtimes.* Mealtimes should be pleasant times for making happy family memories. If you need to reprimand your children, save it for later.
- *Don't become a "mealtime-manners cop."* Yes, you want to teach your children the proper way to eat, but family meals aren't the times to harp on what they're doing wrong. Point out when a child is doing the right thing; resist focusing on his or her mistakes.

- *Be sure everyone participates.* It's easier to create family meals when everyone helps. Divide up mealtime chores as well as privileges. For example, whoever sets the table says grace, or whoever clears the table chooses the topic of conversation.

Make Dietary Changes Gradually

Don't expect to totally revamp your family's eating habits overnight—especially your children's habits. As I mentioned earlier, when Kate and Scott were teens, Barb and I got very serious about nutrition very quickly. However, we made the mistake of trying to change them at our pace rather than at a family pace. I still remember Kate calling Barb's new cooking plan "the Diet of Death!" She wasn't about to withdraw from bad fats and bad sugars so quickly!

We laugh now when we remember those days, but our children had begun to become addicted to some really bad foods. And as you know, addictions, or very strong preferences, can be difficult to change. Food preferences and tastes are developed early in life, mostly during early and middle childhood. Once they are established, they are hard to break. So it's important for me to repeat this: The earlier you encourage healthy food choices for your children, the better.

Changing too much, too fast, can get in the way of dietary success. Begin to remedy excesses or deficiencies by making small changes that, over time, will add up to good, lifelong eating habits. For example, instead of changing instantly from full-fat milk to skim milk, like we tried to do at first, start with 2 percent milk (or a fifty-fifty mixture of full-fat and 2 percent milk). After a few weeks, mix 2 percent and 1 percent (to get 1.5 percent) milk. A few weeks later, change to 1 percent milk. Then, mix skim and 1 percent together for a few weeks. After a few months, you'll have the children drinking skim milk. (I must admit, however, that Barb was a bit sneaky about the gradual milk transition. She kept the lower-fat milk in the full-fat milk container. Our children—until they read this—never knew.)

UNDERSTANDING THE NEED FOR GOOD NUTRITION

We've explored several lifestyle changes we parents can make to improve our family's eating habits and our children's health. While these steps can help, they're only part of the nutritional health picture. The other part of the picture is the foods our children eat.

It's a shocking statistic, but fewer than 1 percent of children in the United States eat what could be considered a healthy diet—the recommended quantities of "good" foods such as whole grains, vegetables, fruits, and low- or no-fat dairy foods. In fact, the CDC has identified a dramatic increase in caloric consumption, particularly from "bad" calories, as the second major cause of weight gain in children and adolescents. One reason for the deteriorating state of our children's nutritional health is that many parents are unaware of their children's need for proper nutrition and don't know which food sources are "good" or "bad."

I don't know about you, but I don't remember having had a course in basic nutrition—not even in medical school! So it shouldn't be surprising that we give our children far more "bad" calories than "good" ones. It wasn't until Barb and I did our own research that I learned to recognize the difference between "good" and "bad" calories. So get ready. I'm going to give you a greatly simplified crash course in "bad" calories—"bad" carbohydrates and "bad" fats—and why they're harmful.

Diets high in "bad" carbohydrates include simple or processed sugars (soft drinks, candy, sweet snack foods) and starches (white rice, white bread, potatoes, most cereals, most pasta, most baked goods). These foods are absorbed quickly and quickly raise the body's blood sugar (glucose) so that the pancreas produces higher-than-normal levels of a hormone called insulin to bring the blood sugar down to normal. At higher levels, insulin increases the accumulation of fat, and excess fat causes insulin resistance, which results in blood sugars being converted to fat and can lead to obesity, type 2 diabetes, heart disease, and blood circulation problems. In addition, "bad" carbohydrates leave the stomach more quickly than do foods that are high in fiber, "good" fats, and proteins, causing hunger to occur earlier than it should.

If this is confusing, consider how it works in real life. A child who eats a sugarcoated cereal soaked in high-fat milk for breakfast is likely to be hungry only two hours later. If he or she is at school, this mid-morning need for a snack is likely to be met by something from a vending machine, which the *New York Times* reports is available to students in 98 percent of American high schools and 43 percent of elementary schools.

Vending machine foods are likely to contain "bad" carbohydrates, "bad" fat, high-calorie carbohydrates (soda, candy bars, bags of cookies, chips). These foods are quickly digested and processed by the child's body so that he or she may be ravenous by lunchtime. For lunch, most schools serve more "bad" foods—highly processed foods, such as pizza, hot dogs, hamburgers, and fries that are high in saturated fat, accompanied by sugar-laden sodas or fruit juices.

Just as there are "bad" carbohydrates, there are "bad" fats as well. "Bad" fats cause hardening of the arteries, heart disease, strokes, and many other health problems. The first group is the *saturated* fats, which are found in milk products (except skim or no-fat milk) and fatty red meat (and to a lesser extent in pork and chicken). Saturated fats should be eliminated as much as possible after the age of two.

A second category of "bad" fats is the *trans fatty acids* (also called trans fats). In 2003, trans fats were listed in the small print on ingredient labels as "partially hydrogenated" oils. New guidelines are now under consideration that may require trans fats to be listed on nutrition labels. Trans fats are found in many margarines, vegetable shortenings, and most snack foods, highly processed foods, and baked goods.

A third category of "bad" fats, called *omega-6 polyunsaturated fatty acids,* should be used very sparingly. They are found in corn oils, cottonseed oils, sunflower oils, and safflower oils, as well as in some soy products. An excessive intake of omega-6 fats may promote inflammatory diseases (such as arthritis and heart disease) and some forms of cancer. The average American child consumes twice the maximum recommended amount of these fats.

Eating so many of the wrong kinds of foods has a disastrous impact on health. United States Department of Agriculture (USDA) data show that the diets of most children are low in many nutrients, especially vitamins E and B6, and the minerals zinc, calcium, and iron. These deficiencies occur because children are eating the foods with low nutritional value that rob them of nutrients and vitamins. Data from a 1998 survey of more than 5,500 American children from birth to nine years of age, when compared to the results of a similar survey from 1994 to 1996, showed a rise in snack and soft-drink consumption and a decline in milk consumption. In the more recent study, snacks contributed about 20 percent of the daily calories consumed! Over the past two decades, soft drink consumption increased 21 percent among two- to five-year-olds and 37 percent among six- to nine-year-olds. The average child or teen now consumes as much as sixty-five gallons of soda each year! No wonder our children aren't getting the nutrition they need!

These nutritional habits have a negative impact on children's health in other ways as well. One study suggested that children who drink too much cola may experience "caffeine-induced" headaches on a daily basis. This high caffeine intake may also rob children of much-needed sleep.

Many parents know some of these facts, but think, *Why not let the children enjoy themselves? After all, heart disease, diabetes, and cancer aren't really a problem until they're older, right?* Wrong! When I was in medical school, researchers from the Louisiana State University School of Medicine began doing autopsies on young adults and children who died unexpectedly or in accidents. What shocked those researchers, even in the 1970s, was the incredible degree of premature atherosclerosis (hardening of the arteries) they found *in teenagers.*

More recent studies indicate that good eating habits and exercise during childhood may prevent many health problems in adulthood. One study, for example, concluded that breast cancer prevention should start in childhood— and certainly no later than puberty. In this study of nearly three hundred girls between the ages of eight and ten, half were given counseling on how to follow a diet low in saturated fat. Five years later, the counseling group was eating consistently less fat and more fiber than the other group. More important, lower levels (reductions up to 30 percent) of hormones suspected in breast cancer development were seen in the counseled group. Researchers believe that lower levels of body fat, plus reduced amounts of these hormones, may reduce breast cancer risk.

It's never too early to teach our children to eat correctly, especially since the habits they develop early in life are likely to continue into adulthood.

A PYRAMID FOR NUTRITIONAL HEALTH

In the 1990s, the USDA developed a food guide pyramid as an easy-to-follow guide to healthy eating. The intent was to encourage Americans to adopt a more balanced diet. However, many researchers and medical professionals are displeased with the nutrition message of this pyramid because they believe it relies too heavily on animal foods and refined grains and places far too little emphasis on heart-healthy fruits and vegetables and "good" fats (yes, there are "good" fats, which I'll discuss shortly).

In response, a number of professionals have developed their own versions of the food guide pyramid. My research has led me to do the same. The pyramid that comes closest to the current science, in my opinion, was developed by researchers from Harvard Medical School, and I've adapted their pyramid into my own recommendations.

The pyramid concept makes it easy for parents to visualize the importance of each kind of food that should be part of a healthy diet, and it makes it easier to see which dietary changes need to be made. So here are the building blocks of nutritional health that I believe will encourage a lifetime of good eating habits for your children. Be aware that the lower levels of the pyramid are the most important!

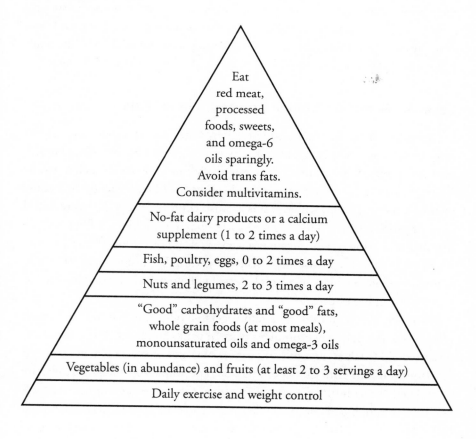

Level 1: Exercise and Weight Control

Many chronic diseases—such as heart attacks, strokes, diabetes, and heart disease—that plague American adults (and increasingly children) are a direct result of obesity and inactivity. The bottom line is that it won't matter how well our children eat if they don't get moving! In chapter 11, I'll share some ideas on family exercise and activity.

Level 2: Vegetables and Fruit

Vegetables and fruits provide essential vitamins, minerals, fiber, and disease-preventing phytochemicals. Research points out the benefits of consuming leafy greens and berries. When making choices, aim for a maximum of color diversity. Every color of fruit and vegetable delivers unique health benefits.

Although five servings a day of fruits and vegetables is the standard recommendation, the more you and your children eat the better. Some researchers now recommend up to nine servings a day for adolescent and adult men (especially African-Americans) and up to seven servings a day for adolescent and adult women in order to reduce the risk of cancer and other age-related diseases.

Level 3: "Good" Carbohydrates and "Good" Fats

I explained earlier about "bad" carbohydrates and fats, but some of our most important foods are "good" carbohydrates and fats. No nutritional health plan is complete without them. Here's why: Whole grain foods such as whole wheat, brown rice, or oatmeal are good sources of fiber, minerals, and some vitamins. Stone-ground whole grains are also good and are quite easily found at most grocery stores. These "good" carbohydrates are high in fiber and are digested more slowly, which causes a slower release of carbohydrates into the bloodstream and keeps insulin levels from getting harmfully high. They also contain numerous phytochemicals believed to help maintain good health and prevent a number of diseases.

The "good" fats found in certain vegetable oils, nuts, fish oil, and many plant foods also deserve a prominent place in your child's diet. These monounsaturated oils (such as olive oils and canola oils) and omega-3 polyunsaturated fats (found in oily fish, canola oil, flax oil, and unhydrogenated soy oils) are considered "heart healthy" because they slow the progression of heart disease and do not raise blood cholesterol levels. The idea of "good" fats is supported by evidence from Mediterranean and Nordic cultures where people consume high amounts of these plant oils and fatty fish, yet have much lower rates of obesity, diabetes, and heart disease than Americans.

Not only are "good" fats beneficial for your child's heart health; problems can result if a child doesn't consume enough of them. Studies have shown that a low-fat diet (low in good *and* bad fats) actually increases a young child's risk of stroke later in life. Before age two, children shouldn't have restrictions on the amount of fat they consume because many fats are crucial to the development of the brain, spinal cord, and nerves. But beginning at age two (and no later than age six), many of the dietary fat recommendations that apply to adults also apply to children.

Level 4: Nuts and Legumes

Nuts provide high-quality protein and come packed with good fats. Even appropriate amounts of peanut butter are a healthy food source as long as it does not contain trans fat (look for the word *hydrogenated* on the label). Multiple studies show that small amounts of nuts on a daily basis help reduce the "bad" cholesterol (called LDL)—or the "lethal" cholesterol.

Legumes are another good source of protein. The fiber in legumes helps control the appetite. Furthermore, studies indicate that they help reduce the risk of heart disease and may even prevent some forms of cancer.

Level 5: Fish, Poultry, and Eggs

Unlike red meat, fish has almost no artery-clogging saturated fat and has a healthy dose of "good" fats. These fats, including the omega-3 fatty acids, help make important hormones that regulate body functions. Meats that are low in saturated fats, such as white meat poultry (chicken and turkey) without the skin, can add good protein to your child's diet with a minimum of "bad" fats. Eggs are also considered to be an excellent source of protein for children. The latest research shows that an egg or two a day is not bad for your child's heart and health. In fact, egg yolks contain two powerful phytochemicals (lutein and zeanxanthin) that promote eye health.

Level 6: Dairy Products or Calcium Supplements

A growing group of nutrition scientists believe, as do I, that it is not necessary to rely solely on dairy foods for calcium or protein once a child reaches the age of three or four. According to research by Katherine Tucker of Tufts University, if we focused more on whole foods, such as whole grains, legumes, and produce, we would create a positive mineral balance and easily meet our children's daily calcium needs. Other good sources of calcium are low-fat yogurt, soy-based products, and calcium-fortified orange juice.

Despite the ease with which calcium needs could be met, the American Academy of Pediatrics warns that children and adolescents in the United States

are not getting enough calcium. Because of this deficiency, the Academy recommends a daily diet that includes milk, yogurt, cheese, and other calcium-
rich foods for children. However, they stress that fat-reduced or fat-free dairy
products (such as skim milk) are fine for older children. For children and adolescents who cannot or will not consume adequate amounts of calcium from
any dietary sources, parents should consider the use of mineral supplements.

Level 7: Eat Certain Foods Sparingly and Consider Multivitamins

I agree with Walter Willett's recommendation to include red meat, butter, white rice, white bread, potatoes, pasta, fried foods, and sweets into one
category at the very tip of the pyramid. These items are to be eaten only
rarely—if at all. Most snack foods fall into this category. Sweets contain
"empty calories" that may contribute to weight gain and diabetes. Keep in
mind that not all scientists buy into the theory that potatoes and pasta are bad
for children, but most agree that loading up on one kind of food (such as
pasta) while shunning other kinds of foods (such as vegetables) is an unhealthy
way to eat.

In addition to the risk of "bad" fats and carbohydrates in this group, there
is a new risk to consider. Researchers in several countries are concerned that
fries, potato chips, other deep-fried foods, and some baked goods contain a
potentially dangerous substance known as acrylamide, which *may* cause cancer in humans. Acrylamide has shown the capability of being passed through
the placenta or through breast milk to a baby. The Food and Drug Administration is working on plans to reduce this substance in foods, but even if acrylamide is shown not to be dangerous, we should still avoid these foods as much
as possible.

Although some experts now recommend a multivitamin for all children—
and 25 to 50 percent of children in the United States take one—the American Academy of Pediatrics recommends that (1) all infants, including those
who are exclusively breast-fed, have a minimum intake of 200 international
units of vitamin D per day, beginning during the first two months of life, and
(2) children who do not drink fluoridated water may need fluoride supplements. Mothers who exclusively breast-feed should also talk to their child's
physician about oral vitamin K.

Most experts believe a daily multivitamin is not necessary for otherwise
healthy children who have a nutritious diet. They believe it is best to try to

meet the daily requirements or recommended daily allowance of nutrients by providing children with a well-balanced diet. I agree with these recommendations. I am concerned that "vitamin popping" may actually encourage poor eating and nutrition habits and cause children whose parents give them a daily vitamin to think they *have* to take a pill every day in order to stay well. Furthermore, vitamins can be expensive, and taking too much of the wrong ones may be harmful. However, children on a poor diet, preterm infants, or children with chronic medical problems may need supplements.

Regardless of how they interpret the principles of good nutrition, most experts give much the same advice: Feed your children a diet high in fruits, vegetables, and whole grain foods; give them more fish and much less red meat; choose low-fat dairy foods (if you include dairy in their diet); and choose vegetable oils and spreads rather than animal fats such as butter. (By the way, you may be thinking, *If your recommendations are so good, why doesn't the USDA consider revising the food pyramid?* The fact is, the food scientists at the USDA are revising their old pyramid and tell me the new pyramid should be ready for publication by 2005.)

The approach you take to your children's nutrition not only is essential to their health today but also will dramatically affect whether they are highly healthy teens, adults, and parents. One group of researchers sums up the essential role nutrition plays in childhood health:

> Recent evidence shows that infancy, toddler, and early childhood years (ages 0 to 6) are perhaps the most important developmental stages for establishing healthy eating and exercise patterns. These patterns can provide optimal growth and cognitive development, and prevent a lifetime of obesity and nutrition-related diseases. If children do not eat the appropriate nutrients and engage in physical activity during these early years, by the time they enter school they may already show signs of cognitive impairment, be overweight or at risk for obesity, and have established eating patterns that result in a lifetime of insufficient intake of milk, fruits and vegetables, and key nutrients, like iron and calcium.

I wholeheartedly agree. Proper nutrition and exercise are areas where most parents can easily take steps to significantly improve the balance in their child's physical wheel.

NUTRITION FOR LITTLE ONES

There is absolutely no question that the very best first food for your child is breast milk. More than thirty years of research has taught us that the Creator has custom-designed a mother's milk to perfectly nourish and to protect a baby from illness. Human milk contains at least a hundred ingredients not found in formula, and we've only begun to understand its many benefits.

In addition to providing nutrition, breast-feeding promotes jaw development in a manner different from bottle-feeding. This may be one of the reasons breast-fed infants tend to have fewer cavities than formula-fed babies and to need fewer orthodontic corrections. During childhood, breast-fed infants have lower rates of hospitalizations, ear infections, colds, diarrhea, rashes, allergies, asthma, sudden infant death syndrome, and childhood lymphoma. When breast-fed babies grow up, they tend to experience less diabetes, hypertension, obesity, allergies, and asthma.

Exclusively breast-fed babies also have fewer infectious illnesses because breast milk contains a mother's infection-fighting antibodies. So breast-fed babies are generally protected from pneumonia, botulism, bronchitis, staphylococcal infections, influenza, ear infections, and German measles. The protection, of course, is not absolute, but the risk for these infections is significantly reduced. Breast-feeding moms continually produce antibodies to illnesses to which they are exposed, and these new antibodies are passed along in their milk.

Nursing appears to have psychological benefits for the baby, too. Psychologists believe that a nursing baby obtains a sense of security from the mother's warmth and presence—a security that does not occur with bottle-feeding. At birth, infants see only about fifteen inches—almost exactly the distance between a nursing baby and its mother's face! Nursing creates an early and intense attachment between the mom and her baby. Studies have shown that babies as young as one week seem to prefer the smell of their own mothers' milk. When nursing pads soaked with breast milk are placed in their cribs, they turn their faces toward the ones that smell like their moms.

The American Academy of Family Physicians and the American Academy of Pediatrics recommend that babies be exclusively breast-fed for at least six months and preferably for twelve months. When a woman cannot, for a variety of medical, emotional, or social reasons, breast-feed, infant formula is the only acceptable alternative. Solid foods can be introduced when a baby is four to six months old. However, it's not considered safe to use cow's milk until a child is a year old or older. Breast-feeding beyond the first year is both healthy and recommended. Increasingly moms are breast-feeding for six months or longer.

Resource Box   *Helpful Hints*

Additions to Infant Formula

Experts disagree about whether certain long-chain polyunsaturated fatty acids (DHA and ARA) should be included in infant formula. My conclusion is that DHA/ARA supplements are not necessary for normal newborns. In addition, the American Academy of Pediatrics does not feel there is enough data to recommend them. You can learn more about this at my website (www.highlyhealthy.net).

What about Baby Foods?

During the time I was writing this book, a television commercial for Gerber Graduates foods questioned whether an older baby who nibbles at the family meals is getting the right nutrition. The commercial showed actress Jane Seymour and her twins as she scolds parents to not "let a milestone become a mistake by starting adult foods too early." She tells parents that their food may not provide all the nutrition their children need.

Gerber is not alone in trying to expand sales in the $4 billion U.S. baby food market. Heinz offers Toddler Cuisine, a line of microwave meals for children from nine months to thirty-six months of age. Mead Johnson Nutritionals' Enfagrow line of fortified snacks is aimed for children up to age four. However, there is no need to stock up on baby foods for older babies. Although these prepackaged foods are convenient, they are not nutritionally necessary, and some experts claim that these "transitional foods" are unhealthy.

William C. Heird, who chairs a March of Dimes panel that is developing food guidelines for children under the age of two, says older babies are better off eating regular food. Dr. Heird, a professor of pediatrics at the Baylor College of Medicine's Children's Nutrition Research Center, is concerned that these food products provide additional calories that will only contribute to the obesity trend.

My own concerns about commercial baby foods, whether for infants or toddlers, are threefold:

1. They may not be as fresh or as healthy as home-prepared foods, especially if you practice good nutritional habits.
2. The predetermined portions may lead you to ignore your child's natural desire to stop eating when full. I've lost count of the number of times I've seen a parent force a baby to finish a jar.
3. Sharing in the family meal, as I discussed earlier, is critical for the development of your child's emotional, social, and spiritual health. Eating at the table with the family, especially after age two, allows your child to get plenty of proper nutrition. Older babies simply need to eat a variety of foods, including dairy products, fruits and vegetables, white meat, and eggs.

Resource Box   *Helpful Hints*

Increasingly, parents are avoiding commercial baby foods and choosing to cook and puree their own fruits and vegetables. I've often recommended *Mommy Made and Daddy Too: Home Cooking for a Healthy Baby and Toddler* by Martha and David Kimmel (with Suzanne Goldenson). Updated information on this book can be found at the www.highlyhealthy.net website.

What's the Truth about Fruit Juices?

Believe it or not, the American Academy of Pediatrics is concerned that parents may be giving their children *too* much fruit juice. Without a doubt, fruit juice can be a healthy part of a child's diet. It is a good source of vitamin C and—if the juice is fortified—calcium. But studies show that infants who drink too much juice may become malnourished if fruit juice replaces human milk or formula in their diet.

Fruit juices are not a replacement for human milk. Fruit juices usually don't contain any significant amount of proteins, fats, minerals, or other vitamins.

Worse, many contain large amounts of simple sugars (the "bad" sugars). When these sugars are consumed in large quantities, the result can be diarrhea, cramps, bloating, and gas. Juice consumption also increases the risk of cavities and tooth decay because fruit drinks or fruit juice "cocktails" include extra sweeteners, artificial flavors, and other ingredients.

Here are the American Academy of Pediatrics' recommendations for fruit juice consumption:

- Fruit juice should not be given to infants younger than six months of age.
- Infants should not get juice from bottles or cups that allow them to drink juice throughout the day.
- Infants should not get fruit juice at bedtime.
- For children ages one to six, juice intake should be limited to four to six ounces per day.
- For children ages seven to eighteen, juice intake should be between eight and twelve ounces a day.
- All children should be encouraged to eat whole fruits.

OF COURSE YOU'LL HAVE QUESTIONS

In a book this size there's no way I can explain everything you need to know about the nutritional needs of highly healthy children. I've only outlined the foundation of healthy childhood nutrition, and now it's up to you to continue the process. In this section I'll address some of the more common questions asked by parents of my young patients.

What If My Child Is a Picky Eater?

This is the most common question I'm asked. Many parents worry that their picky eaters aren't eating as much as they should. Yet even the pickiest eaters who seem to have a relatively low food intake grow at normal rates. Why? There is great variation in how and what different children—even those of the same size, same gender, or same family—eat. Some children have smaller appetites, while others are just plain finicky. Children's appetites also tend to fluctuate as they grow. Children increase their food consumption considerably as they enter the growth spurts associated with puberty. Until then, a child's appetite may be unpredictable.

As frustrating as a child's picky eating habits may be, keep in mind that you, too, may have foods you like and dislike. In general, youngsters outgrow these food preferences without any harm to their physical well-being. In most cases, go along with your child's wishes, as long as he or she likes enough foods to achieve a balanced diet and to grow within normal ranges.

What If My Child or Teenager Wants to Be a Vegetarian?

For most children, not only is a vegetarian diet safe, it may even be highly healthy. Dieticians do have three concerns with regard to vegetarian children, however:

- *Vitamin B-12 deficiency.* Vitamin B-12 is found primarily in meat, eggs, and milk. Fortunately, parents can find B-12-fortified cereals, soy milk, and veggie burgers, as well as inexpensive oral B-12 supplements.
- *Risk of deficiency of minerals such as iron, calcium, and zinc.* Although these minerals are present in vegetables like kale, broccoli, and spinach, animal sources of these minerals are absorbed better. Food producers are now beginning to add mineral supplements to orange juice, soy milk, and cereals.
- *Risk of not getting sufficient calories for growth.* Vegetables are far less calorie-dense than meat or dairy foods, which is why we adults can eat so many of them without concern. When babies or toddlers are put on a vegetarian diet, we need to ensure that they have enough calories, especially the essential fatty acids that are necessary for brain and nerve development. These fatty acids are found in vegetable oils, nuts, seeds, margarine, and fish oils.

Worries about protein deficiency among children who eat a vegetarian diet have been shown not to be a concern, especially if these children eat eggs and drink milk. Even if children avoid eggs and milk, foods such as whole grain rice, beans, soybeans, and wheat can provide plenty of protein.

What's the Truth about Pesticides?

As parents, we must know the truth about pesticides and take steps to protect our children. They face a much greater health risk from pesticides than we do. Children may be more vulnerable because their internal organs are still developing and maturing. In addition, their metabolic and immune systems are less likely than those of an adult to provide protection. Children are also vulnerable because they typically consume much larger quantities of milk, applesauce, apple juice, and orange juice per pound of body weight than do teens or adults.

Thankfully, the risk of pesticide exposure is already quite small, and you can dramatically reduce the risk by using the following food preparation practices:

- *Wash and scrub.* Wash and scrub thoroughly all fresh fruits and vegetables under running water. (Running water is much more effective than soaking.) Doing so helps remove bacteria, traces of chemicals, and dirt from the surface—especially if you don't buy organic fruits and vegetables.
- *Peel and trim.* Peel fruits and vegetables when possible to reduce dirt, bacteria, or pesticides. Also discard the outer leaves of leafy vegetables. In addition, trim fat from meat and the skin from poultry and fish, because pesticide residues can collect in fat.
- *Select a variety of foods.* Eating a variety of foods from a variety of sources protects your children by providing a better mix of nutrients and reducing the likelihood of exposure to a single pesticide.
- *Consider buying organically grown foods for your family.* To legally carry the label "organically grown," food must be grown and processed using no synthetic fertilizers or pesticides. Pesticides derived from natural sources (biological pesticides, for example) are sometimes used in producing organically grown food. Many supermarkets now stock organic products, though these foods may be as much as 20 to 100 percent more expensive than nonorganic varieties. So the "wash and peel" methods described above should provide adequate protection for budget-conscious families.

Resource Box   **Helpful Hints**

Pesticide Exposure

Fruits and vegetables with the highest pesticide exposure are peaches, apples, strawberries, nectarines, pears, cherries, red raspberries, imported grapes, spinach, bell peppers, celery, potatoes, and hot peppers. I recommend that you either carefully wash and peel these fruits and vegetables before eating or that you consider buying organically grown varieties.

Does It Really Matter How Much or How Fast My Child Eats?

Absolutely! Studies have shown that children and teens feel just as full—no matter whether their food portion is small, average, or super-size. This is especially true if they take more time to eat. So when you and your children eat as a family, when you talk and laugh together, when you take time with each other, you increase your time together and reduce the possibility of overeating (provided you don't add more food to your plate!).

Did you know the recommended serving of cooked meat for an adult is three ounces, similar in size to a deck of playing cards? A medium piece of fruit is one serving. It doesn't take much nutritious food to fill you up and provide the healthy nutrition you and your children need. So if you keep your children's portions (and your own) reasonable, it's much easier for them to eat the foods you want them to eat and thus to stay healthy.

Many of us during our childhood days were taught or cajoled to "clean our plates"—to finish every bite, even if we were full. Given current information, I'm sure you see the wisdom of serving smaller portions and not worrying about whether your children clean their plates. Teaching them to eat slowly and to stop once they begin to feel full is wise parenting.

But, you may be muttering to yourself, *if I do this, they'll be back in the kitchen for a snack in an hour or two.*

"Great!" Just have healthy or nutritious snacks ready for them—a sliced apple or peeled orange, fruit and yogurt, a soy or yogurt shake, a whole grain snack. Leave the ready-made, high-fat, high-sugar snacks out of the picture.

Not only do most adults and children eat too much, but we eat too fast as well. Even when we have time to relax and enjoy our food, we still tend to inhale our meals. Physiologically, it takes twenty to twenty-five minutes before a child's brain (and yours, too) receives the "full" signal from the stomach. If your children eat quickly, they may have eaten too much food by the time the "full" signal reaches the brain and turns off the hunger signal. We all know how much food a child can shovel into his or her mouth in twenty minutes! We can help our children eat more slowly by slowing down ourselves. Here are some suggestions:

- *Use small plates.* Small plates help you and your child gain control over your portion sizes. Small plates trick your children's minds—and yours—into thinking they've eaten more than they actually have. In one study, some people were given food on a small plate; others received food on a medium or large plate. After they were done eating, most people in all three groups felt the same degree of fullness. (The "small plate" strategy will not work, however, if your children consume three or four helpings.)

- *Start your meal with a healthy vegetable soup, fruit dish, or salad.*
- *Serve your meal in courses.* When everyone has finished the first course, clear the table and wait three to five minutes before serving the second course.
- *Encourage your children to taste their food.* Having children describe the taste of food slows them down. Most of them don't even think about taste.
- *Encourage your children, when old enough, to put food on their own plates.* A study in 2003 found that when children serve themselves, they actually eat less than when a parent serves them and still get an appropriate amount of food.
- *Encourage your children to chew each bite at least ten times and to count to ten between bites, or have them place their fork or spoon on the table between each bite.*

Now, I don't suggest being legalistic about these recommendations (after all, your home is not a military academy!), but if you practice these techniques as a family, you will significantly increase the amount of time you spend at the table. Just think of all the talking your family will enjoy as you dine together!

Are Food Allergies For Real?

Experts tell us that only about 3 percent of children are affected by food allergies, but the percentage is rapidly rising. According to the Food Allergy Network, about one hundred people die nationwide each year from allergic reactions to food. Among children, allergies to milk, eggs, and peanuts are most common. Other common allergens include wheat, soy, tree nuts, fish, and shellfish. About one child in 150 has a peanut allergy, which may be one of the most dangerous childhood food allergies.

Please note that I'm discussing true allergies that result in an allergic reaction in the body's immune system; I'm *not* talking about a sensitivity to food— which is not a true allergic reaction but occurs much more frequently. True food allergies can cause a number of symptoms, including diarrhea, cramping, vomiting, hives or eczema on the skin, wheezing, coughing, or swelling of the lips or tongue. Severe reactions may be combined, and a combination of two or more types of these symptoms—or one symptom that's life-threatening—is called an *anaphylactic reaction* that should be treated immediately with the EpiPen (auto-injectors of epinephrine) and Benadryl (an oral antihistamine), followed by a visit to the emergency room.

Resource Box   Helpful Hints

The Food Allergy and Anaphylaxis Network (FAAN) sells trainer EpiPens and provides cards that teach people how to read food labels. Parents are also encouraged to get in touch with the Food Allergy Initiative (FAI) organization, which is useful in supporting research and public policy. You can learn more about the EpiPen and about the FAI at www.highlyhealthy.net.

Testing for suspected food allergies can potentially prevent a life-threatening allergic or anaphylactic reaction. There are two ways to test for a food allergy. Doctors usually conduct a blood test for children under the age of two or a skin test for older children. Both tests have disadvantages. Skin tests can return false positives (indicating an allergy when there is none). Blood tests are invasive and are only as good as the lab that does the testing. Many doctors do both—generally the skin test first. Interpreting the test, however, is an art rather than a science.

Before testing, parents need to keep an accurate food diary for two weeks. Most allergists recommend eliminating the suspected food for two weeks. Parents need to learn how to read food labels so the suspected food can be removed from their children's diet completely. If, after the elimination, the symptoms stop, then the allergy is determined. Children, however, are often allergic to more than one food. Once a child's allergy is confirmed, a doctor will usually prescribe at least three EpiPens and Benadryl. You can learn more about food allergies at my website (www.highlyhealthy.net).

Chapter Six

Provide Adequate Protection

When Scott was just three years old, Barb asked me to watch him while I barbecued hamburgers in our backyard. In what seemed like only a few moments, she came outside and asked, "Where's Scott?"

I looked around, and Scott was nowhere to be seen. We did not have a fenced yard, and he was gone! I can't begin to describe the overwhelming feelings of disbelief, horror, and embarrassment I felt. After a frantic search, we found him, but I still get chills up and down my spine thinking of that day.

The thought of a child being harmed in any way absolutely terrifies most parents. Headline-making stories of abductions, accidents, murder, and abuse stoke the fires of parental fear on a regular basis. Researchers tell us that today's parents view the hazards in our culture as "a source of constant worry, posing an even tougher problem than household finances or lack of family time!" Believing that our culture is inhospitable and even dangerous for children, parents feel they must be on guard constantly to protect their children. For many parents, "there are just too many dangers, too many temptations, and too many harmful influences for them to relax."

I understand their concern. There is nothing easy about raising children in today's world. Roughly three-quarters (76 percent) of parents in one recent national survey realize how hard this job is, and more than half of them (53 percent) believe they are doing a worse job than their parents. Yet nurturing children to become healthy physically, emotionally, relationally, and spiritually is one of the most important responsibilities God gives us.

The word *nurture* comes from the agrarian term *brood,* which implies safety and security. The image conveyed is that of parent birds holding their chicks under their wings, providing comfort and safety. The folk story about a ranger walking through a park after a forest fire illustrates this beautifully. The ranger came across a dead bird at the base of a tree, petrified in ash. Curious, he poked at the bird with his walking stick. Immediately three small chicks scurried out from under the bird's wing!

As parents, our self-sacrificing job of providing security and safety from the dangers of our world is essential to our children's well-being. Let me tell you about a time when my daughter, Kate, reminded me of how important the perception of safety is in the life of a highly healthy child.

Kate returned home after taking a weekend trip with her Girl Scout troop. She had enjoyed a great time hiking, camping, swimming, cooking, and laughing. After showering, she came into the living room where I was reading.

"Is your lap available for a girl?" she asked, smiling at me, knowing how special it was for us to talk when she was sitting on my lap.

"Of course," I said. She plopped down as I put my book aside, sat quietly for a moment, and sighed deeply. I waited for a moment before inquiring, "What's up?"

"Oh, nothing," she replied, as she snuggled into my hug. "I just feel so *safe* here."

PROTECTION BEGINS AT HOME

As parents, we can't shield our children from all of the what-ifs of living in a dangerous world. I remember how Barb and I struggled to know how to protect our children. On one hand, we wanted to prevent harm and unnecessary pain; on the other hand, we knew they needed to become independent, so we didn't want to be overprotective and stifle their development.

We realized we could identify threats to our children and take practical actions to reduce the risks, but the most effective protection would be to teach our children how to protect themselves. We wanted to raise them with the skills and values they needed in order to choose to do what is right—which included teaching our children to refuse peers or adults who pressed them to participate in questionable, dangerous, immoral, or illegal acts. Training our children to protect themselves begins at home with the parent-child relationship.

We Protect Our Children by Building
Strong Relationships with Them

Preparing for life in an unsafe world begins when a child feels secure in his or her immediate home environment. We always wanted our children to echo that sigh of feeling safe and comfortable, as Kate did that day in my lap. Child psychologists confirm that protection and loving supervision are necessary in order for children to become highly healthy. So it's especially important for preschool children to play and learn in a home environment in which they feel safe, secure, comfortable, and loved.

Children want to feel loved and to be listened to when they share their concerns. In a loving home, a child feels more comfortable talking about likes and dislikes, friends, school, and feelings and is more likely to turn to his or her parents to discuss fears and concerns. But let me be clear: This kind of home environment requires parents to make a significant time investment. As I explained earlier, quality time with a child occurs *only* during quantity time.

Parents cannot provide quality time if they are not present, and many parents tell me they regret not spending more time with their children. Jenny was one such parent. She had a successful career and seemed to have a successful marriage. She and her husband went on expensive vacations and placed their children, from the very earliest ages, in the best day care centers. When Jenny's career required more travel, she hired a nanny to care for her children at night and on weekends. When I questioned her about the small amount of time she was spending with her children, she patted my arm and stated confidently, "There will be time later, Dr. Larimore. Don't worry."

"Jenny," I scolded, "your children need you *now* more than they will later. No one can be the mother to them that you can be. They need *you*." She furrowed her brow and was quiet for a moment. Then she said she would think about it.

Several months later, Jenny had a routine physical and had some blood tests done. I called Jenny to come back to my office because her blood tests showed some abnormal results. Worried, she and her husband canceled all plans and rushed over to my office. The diagnosis? An uncommon and very dangerous form of leukemia.

That night I admitted Jenny to the hospital. When I visited Jenny and her husband that night, they seemed almost jovial. "Friends tell us that most cases of leukemia can be healed with treatment. So let's get started!" Jenny exclaimed.

I didn't want to diminish her hope, but I also needed Jenny and her husband to understand the very poor prognosis she was facing. We had a long talk, followed by a special time of prayer together.

Jenny never went home again. She died in the hospital ten days later.

Two nights before she died we talked about her children, and she confided, "If only . . ." I tried to reassure her, but she was right. If only . . .

I hope I can help you realize how important your actual presence for significant periods of time is in the life of each of your children. Maybe you've made decisions that haven't fostered strong relationships with your children. Maybe you, like Jenny, have put off spending time with your children. Or maybe you're just beginning to make changes in this area. Whatever your situation is, *now* is the time to start doing what's right for you and your family. The decisions you make today can influence the health of your children, your grandchildren, and your great-grandchildren.

Resource Box   **Helpful Hints**

Ways to Build Strong Relationships with Your Children

It's not easy to create a home environment that nurtures strong parent-child relationships, especially if you never experienced such an environment yourself. Here are a few things Barb and I did to encourage strong relationships with our children:

- At least once a day (and usually far more often) we would show our children—through hugs, words, gestures, notes, and occasional small gifts—how much we loved them.
- We worked to build our children's esteem and confidence by going out of our way to find them doing things right and then recognizing and applauding their accomplishments.
- We worked on *really* listening to our children—which meant turning off the television or radio, putting down what we were doing, and looking into our children's eyes and listening to them.
- We encouraged our children to be involved in activities outside the home but tried to limit their activity to one

> sport or hobby at a time. Time at home was healthier than time spent almost anywhere else.
>
> - As our children grew in age and wisdom, we respected their need for privacy and their growing independence, but we never relinquished our responsibility to stay involved with them and to supervise them.
> - Both Barb and I found mature mentors who shared their experiences with us, gave us advice, and held us accountable when we faced difficult problems in protecting our children.
>
> Talk with your spouse about these ideas, come up with some of your own, and put into practice those you like best. Remind each other of these relationship-builders daily.

WE PROTECT OUR CHILDREN THROUGH DISCIPLINE—SETTING SAFE LIMITS TO BE OBEYED

Building strong relationships with our children in an atmosphere of love and openness is an essential step toward ensuring their safety, but it's just the first step. Children also need parental guidance and enforced boundaries if they are to stay safe and healthy. It's vital that your love and authority be demonstrated through discipline from the earliest stages of your child's development so that he or she will learn how to make wise, safe decisions.

The term *discipline* has several meanings. The dictionary's first definition of the noun *discipline* is "training that develops self-control, character, or orderliness and efficiency." Yet many parents use the word *discipline* in the same way they use the word *punishment*—which is the last meaning of the word. The verb *to discipline* is defined similarly. The first definition is "to subject to discipline; to instruct or educate; to prepare by instruction; to train." The second definition is "to chastise; to punish."

Discipline is absolutely necessary in the life of a highly healthy child. Its most important purpose is to help a child learn to function in a highly healthy fashion. The Michigan Psychological Association says, "The purpose of discipline is to teach our children appropriate behavior so they may get along with others and live effectively in the world. It involves guiding children to make wise decisions about their conduct and gradually allowing them to accept the responsibility for their choices. Providing direction, correcting undesirable behavior, and teaching acceptable responses is an important part of being a parent." Discipline requires, on occasion, punishment. But more important, discipline involves defining protective boundaries and helping children learn that there will almost always be consequences for breaching those boundaries.

Six Keys to Protecting Our Children through Discipline

We parents don't come equipped with the skills we need to be great parents. We must learn them, and to learn them we need a teacher. During the past twenty-five years, Dr. James Dobson has become well-known for teaching parents loving and effective ways to raise their children. Barb and I devoured his books as we raised Kate and Scott. Many evenings just before going to bed, we'd read part of a chapter from *Dare to Discipline* or *The Strong-Willed Child*. From Dr. Dobson's writings, we learned six keys to shaping a healthy child. I'd like to share them with you:

1. Define the Boundaries before They Are Enforced

Establish reasonable expectations and boundaries, and communicate them *in advance.* Children have the right to know what is and what is not acceptable behavior *before* they are held responsible for keeping those rules. Parents who define the boundaries will virtually eliminate the overwhelming sense of injustice children feel when they are corrected for behavior they didn't know was unacceptable. If you haven't *clearly* explained a boundary to your child, don't enforce it!

Barb and I had certain rules for everyone in our family: Everyone always wore a seat belt in the car; it was not acceptable to interrupt when another person was talking; we went to church together every Sunday. Not only did we hold our children accountable for these behaviors; we allowed our children to hold us accountable as well.

2. Avoid Making Impossible Demands

Impossible demands put children in a terrible position in which they cannot win and will invariably be damaged in the process. Although it's wise and healthy for us to encourage our children to do the very best they can—to push them to do things in an excellent manner—it is our responsibility to be absolutely sure our children are capable of doing what we expect. For example, it is inappropriate to correct a two-year-old for wetting the bed involuntarily at night. Most children are not toilet trained by twenty-four months of age. Likewise, to fuss at a child for not getting an "A" when he or she is not capable of greater academic accomplishment will only break the child's spirit.

Children cannot be highly healthy if they live under the thumb of a perfectionist tyrant. There is no way out of the turmoil perfectionism causes. In response, children tend either to rebel or to escape—both of which are damaging. Rebellion and escape move children away from the protection they need and prevent them from becoming highly healthy.

3. Distinguish between Willful Defiance and Childish Irresponsibility

I still remember the first time I heard Dr. Dobson teach that children should never be punished for behavior that is not willfully defiant. It really hit home to me. When Kate, age six, would forget to put her dirty clothes in the laundry hamper, or when Scott, age three, would leave a blanket in the living room, I needed to realize that these behaviors were normal for children of their ages. These were acts of childish irresponsibility, not willful defiance. When a child willfully chooses to rebel, it is appropriate for parents to allow the child to experience well-defined consequences. However, childish irresponsibility should be handled patiently with careful instruction.

4. When Defiantly Challenged, Respond with Confident Decisiveness

Once children understand what is expected, parents need to hold them accountable to behave accordingly. A highly healthy child must learn that breaching a boundary is potentially harmful and that such a breach will always have consequences.

When nose-to-nose confrontations happen, it is extremely important to know ahead of time what you will do. Dr. Dobson warns that children will make it clear that they're looking for a fight, and you would be wise not to disappoint them. *Nothing* is more destructive to your efforts to provide a foundation of protection for your child than to fail to teach or discipline your child during these struggles. Children need to see us as secure and confident parents who will quickly and lovingly allow them to experience consequences for their willful defiance.

5. Reassure and Teach after the Confrontation Is Over

After each incident of willful defiance, regardless of the correction required, our children need reassurance that we love them. After punishment, when they've calmed down, we can open our arms—and our laps—and hold them close. We can tell them how much we love them. We must, however, be sure to emphasize why they were corrected or punished and remind them how they can avoid correction or punishment in the future. These special moments build love and respect while also teaching the consequences of failing to follow established rules.

6. Let Love Be Our Guide

Discipline should always be administered in love. *Always!* If we are angry, we should not administer discipline right then. An angry parent needs a time-out!

Our objective as parents is to shape the wills of our children during their earliest years. Discipline, when properly applied, is training a child to recognize and respect the boundaries that are essential to protection. Whether we use positive reinforcement, correcting language, warnings, time-outs, loss of rewards or privileges, or the occasional mild spanking, we need to know which tools to use when. Wise parents will seek to understand the physical and emotional characteristics of their children and match their teaching and discipline to each child's individual needs.

Age-Appropriate Discipline

The need for discipline and the discipline tools that are appropriate to use change as a child matures, and parents have often asked me which types of discipline are appropriate for children of various ages.

During the earliest months, children need security, affection, and warmth. They need to be fed when hungry and kept clean and dry. They need to be held and loved and to hear the soothing voices of their parents. No direct punishment is necessary or appropriate for children under seven months of age. Yet I've known parents who have swatted infants for wiggling while they were being diapered or spanked four-month-old babies for crying at night. These responses are horribly wrong. Babies are simply incapable of not doing these activities. They are not being willfully disobedient; they are simply behaving normally.

When children begin to test parental authority at ages eight months to fourteen months, discipline must be done carefully and gently. Often distraction or diversion may be all that is needed to turn a child's attention in the right direction. When confrontations occur, teach your child by firm persistence, not by punishment. These confrontations will be minor and infrequent, but they mark the beginning of future struggles, so your response is important.

As children approach the age of two, if they aren't frequently saying no, they will. Yet even at this age, mistakes and accidents occur more frequently than willful disobedience. When disobedience occurs, mild forms of punishment such as time-outs or verbal correction often work. When these fail, however, spanking can be considered. I say *considered* because I agree with many experts who teach that spanking is *never* appropriate before eighteen months to twenty-four months and is usually not needed until after twenty-four months of age.

Behavioral control is vitally important in nurturing a highly healthy child, and spanking is necessary to achieve this goal with many children—especially between the ages of two and six. There are too few disciplinary measures for young children to completely exclude spanking from the parents' repertoire. When mild spankings are managed properly, they will not produce harmful emotional or psychological effects. But spanking is not appropriate for every child or at every age, and in many situations it is unnecessary.

Resource Box   *Helpful Hints*

Many parents are confused, and understandably so, about the pros and cons of spanking. Let's see what the experts say.

Conferees at a 1996 scientific conference on spanking defined it as "(1) physically non-injurious, (2) intended to modify behavior, and (3) administered with an opened hand to the extremities or buttocks." They agreed that a mild spanking could make other disciplinary measures more effective in preschoolers with behavior problems.

However, not all experts agree with using the hand to spank. Dr. James Dobson recommends using a neutral object such as a switch or paddle "because the hand should be seen as an object of love—to hold, hug, pat, and caress." He further address the fears of those who see the use of a neutral object as tantamount to child abuse: "I understand their concern, especially in cases when a parent believes 'might makes right' or loses her temper and harms the child. That is why adults must always maintain a balance between love and control, regardless of the method by which they administer disciplinary action."

Diana Baumrind and Elizabeth Owens, psychologists and highly respected researchers on the subject of nonabusive spanking, presented powerful evidence to the 2001 meeting of the American Psychological Association that spanking is *not* harmful when done the right way and in the proper context.

When researchers say spanking is bad for children, they are *not* referring to mild spanking as I define it. They are targeting studies that include not only children who are nonabusively spanked, but also children who *are* abusively spanked and children who are abused in other ways. No wonder these studies show harm! Harsh and abusive physical discipline in the family has been linked to a wide variety of negative outcomes such as poor school performance, poor peer relations, high noncompliance, and delinquency. So parents who lose their tempers or are prone to violence should not use spanking as a disciplinary tool.

Not one well-designed scientific study shows that appropriate nonabusive spanking by a loving parent will breed any type of violence or other negative behaviors in children. When administered appropriately, spanking can be a valuable disciplinary tool. Mild nonabusive spanking is not only effective in itself, but children who have been spanked cooperate better with milder discipline, rendering further spanking and other forms of punishment less necessary.

Can spanking be misused? Absolutely! But so can time-outs and verbal lashings. Should spanking be one of our last resorts as parents? Yes! We parents should vary our response to the particular misbehavior and administer punishment in a way that will be effective for a particular child's temperament.

After age two, children still tend to make many innocent mistakes. They spill things, lose things, damage things, eat almost anything they can get in their mouths, fall off things, explore things, and flush things. While a sense of humor may be one of the most useful parenting tools during these years, these are also the years when parents must begin instilling obedience and respect for authority. If we fail to teach our children to obey and to have a healthy respect for authority, we'll leave them vulnerable to harmful influences.

Parents must remember, however, that the seeds of disrespect and rebellion can take root in a child who does not feel completely loved, secure, and accepted. To overemphasize love and forget to teach obedience can result in disrespect and contempt; to be overly authoritarian and oppressive can result in children feeling unloved and even hated. The goal is for moms and dads to balance love and training, mercy and fairness, warmth and firmness, and tenderness and jurisdiction.

If you've done your job as a parent, the foundation of lifelong protection has been laid by the time your child reaches age nine to twelve. During these preteen years, you can begin to allow more freedom and independent decision making. The overall objective of discipline during these years is to continue teaching your children that their decisions and actions have inevitable consequences.

How does one go about connecting behavior with consequences? By allowing children to experience a reasonable amount of pain when they behave irresponsibly. When our son, Scott, missed the school bus as a result of his irresponsibility, he could either walk the mile to school or wait until it was convenient for his mother or me to take him—and experience the consequences of an unexcused tardiness or absence. If Kate forgot her lunch money, she'd have to borrow money or skip the meal that day.

Every passing year should bring fewer rules, less direct discipline, and more independence because your child has been taught to—and is able to— make wiser, safer choices. As a child becomes more responsible, parents should see much less, if any, need for physical punishment. I agree with the experts who teach that spanking should never (or only very rarely) occur after six to eight years of age. For preteens, physical punishment (as well as excessive verbal castigating) is more likely to be harmful than helpful.

PROTECTING OUR CHILDREN FROM A HOSTILE WORLD

As I wrote this chapter, random shootings were taking place in the Washington, D.C., area. Frightened parents shielded their children as they accompanied them into schools. Schools stopped sending children outside for recess and canceled sports events. Parents and children across the country were feeling a similar kind of fear and anxiety to what they experienced after the September 11 terrorist attacks. In addition, a flurry of media reports highlighted horrifying child abduction and murder cases, as well as the sexual abuse of children by priests or pastors. Even closer to home, children are at risk from other children who are bullies at school or in their neighborhoods. The tentacles of a hostile world even reach into our homes through electronic media such as television and the Internet. No wonder parents and children feel anxious and even fearful!

Although this world fights our efforts to raise highly healthy children, we parents can help our children respond to a hostile world in healthy ways. We must first recognize the impact of traumatic world events on our children. Robert Brooks, a child psychologist at Harvard Medical School, says, "It's important for parents to be aware that children are seeing these events on the news, . . . and that can be scary to any child." You can reassure your children by letting them know that it is highly unlikely that such events would ever happen in your neighborhood, but it's equally important *not* to say that they *cannot* happen. Sadly, it's just not true that it can't happen—no matter where you live.

If your children are afraid, the following ideas adapted from child psychologist Sam Goldstein may prove helpful:

- Don't belittle your children's fears or try to talk them out of how they feel. Listen very carefully, and ask questions such as, "What is bothering you?" or, "How have you been feeling about all this news?" or, "What troubles you the most about these events?"
- Reflect back to your child what you're hearing. You might say, "Are you telling Mommy that this news is scaring you?" Let your child explain, and be sure you keep at it until you understand what he or she is trying to say.
- If you say, "There's no reason to worry," you may appear not to be listening to your child's concerns.
- Ask what you can do to help your child worry less. You might even offer some suggestions. For example, sleeping in your young child's room for a few nights might comfort him or her.
- If necessary, prepare a readiness plan to help youngsters feel more secure. Make sure your child knows telephone numbers and family procedures.

- Realize that each child will react differently. Some may aggressively act out and play shooting games, while others may cling to you. Teens may seem more self-assured but may try to seize an opportunity to talk things out with parents.

By opening up the lines of communication with your child, you can steer him or her toward a realistic perception of potential threats and a healthy response to fear and anxiety. But remember, it takes time and a safe family environment for this to happen. In our family, these times occurred most frequently during dinner or during quiet moments before bedtime.

Guarding against Abduction and Abuse

Many parents harbor great fears that their children will be abducted and abused or perhaps even murdered. In a recent survey, nearly 76 percent of parents voiced this concern, and half of them worried *a lot* about this possibility. Yet the odds of a child being abducted are very low. Although no one can guarantee it won't happen, parents are not helpless in guarding against such crimes. The following simple rules dramatically reduce the threat of an abduction:

- Know where your children are—or should be—at all times.
- Know your children well. Talk to them frequently. Let them know they can safely share their troubles and concerns with you.
- Teach your children not to wander off when you're in public places, even places you visit frequently. A child who actively participates with you (pushing the shopping cart or placing items in it, for example) is more likely to stay with you.
- Know your children's friends, as well as their siblings and parents. Encourage your children to bring their friends home so you can meet them. Talk to the parents of your children's friends on a regular basis.
- Virtually all abductions of children are by people they know—very often they are family members, close friends, or neighbors. Carefully choose the people you allow to spend time with your children. When your children return home from outings, ask questions about what they did and how they felt about it—which gives them an opportunity to express their concerns or fears.
- Teach your children how to get help. They should know how to call 911 and how to contact other people who can help them.

- Teach your children to be wise and to be wary around people they do not know.
- Remember that you will always be your child's most important educator.

In addition to concerns regarding abduction, many parents of young children (63 percent) are very concerned that their children could suffer physical or sexual abuse in day care. Many of the safeguards with regard to abduction also apply to preventing abuse, and parents can find entire books on the subject. Here are a few additional suggestions to consider:

- Whenever possible, screen (with at least a personal interview) *anyone* who will be in close relationship with your child, such as a day care worker, church youth group worker, and so on. Ask if a background check has been done. If not, ask questions of the supervising staff and other parents of children who are participating.
- Be sure you have the right (and understand that you have an obligation) to visit the facility or activity with no advance warning. When you visit, do any of your radars go off? If so, get your child out of there!
- Learn the signs and symptoms of child abuse.
- Always talk with your children after they participate in activities where they've been away from you. Listen for clues that something isn't right.

Resource Box   **Helpful Hints**

Signs and Symptoms of Child Abuse

The signs and symptoms of child abuse can be tricky to sort out. If you have any concerns, be sure to discuss them immediately with your child's physician or call your local police department, sheriff's department, or mental health facility.

If you prefer to talk to folks from outside your local area, you can call Childhelp USA Child Abuse Hotline at 1-800-4-A-CHILD. In addition, you can call and speak to a counselor at Focus on the Family at 1-800-A-FAMILY.

A number of websites provide excellent information on recognizing and dealing with child abuse; you can access these via my website (www.highlyhealthy.net).

When it comes to abuse, your relationship with your child is a tremendous protection to his or her health, although it certainly isn't foolproof. The more your child knows that you are his or her biggest fan and most vigilant guardian, the more likely it is that your child will tell you when he or she feels uncomfortable or unsafe.

Note: It's crucial for parents to protect their children from sexual abuse and harm, premarital sex, and sexually transmitted diseases. However, I'm not discussing the topic in this book for several reasons. First, it would require more space than I have available here, and I'll cover it extensively in my forthcoming book *The Highly Healthy Teen.* Second, many of the principles discussed in this book for improving emotional, relational, and spiritual health will help protect your child from this threat. In anticipation of the publication of *The Highly Healthy Teen,* I've included information on this topic on my website at www.highlyhealthy.net.

THE TRUTH ABOUT BULLYING

Debbie's mom brought her into my office because of changes in her sleep patterns, appetite, weight, and mood. After taking a complete medical history, physical exam, and appropriate laboratory work, I determined that twelve-year-old Debbie was depressed. Although depression is becoming more common in teens, there was no family history of depression, and I couldn't identify a cause. Rather than quickly writing a prescription, I spent a few minutes talking to Debbie alone. I asked questions and listened. Then I asked, "Debbie, what's the hardest thing about going to school?"

Her eyes immediately misted up, and she looked down at her feet. I was quiet for a few moments as she wept. Gently, I touched her arm. "Debbie, you can tell me."

"You won't tell *anyone,* will you, Dr. Walt?"

"Not without your permission."

Debbie shared a story of physical and mental abuse that was being heaped on her daily by a small group of girls at her school. Debbie was terrified. She feared for her life. No wonder she was depressed! She didn't need a prescription; she needed protection.

Far too many children, like Debbie, are bullied. As a result they are agitated, frustrated, and desperate for a way out. As parents, we need to take bullying very seriously. My colleague Bob Smithouser clearly describes the serious nature of bullying: "Bullying is not horseplay. It's not impish sarcasm or an isolated fistfight. Bullying is deliberately hurtful behavior repeated over time against a victim unable to defend himself or herself. It can be broadly characterized as either physical, verbal, or indirect (spreading rumors, intentional exclusion from social groups, etc.)."

Bullying can have a terrible impact. As many as 86 percent of children in the United States say they've been bullied, and research shows that children consider the death of someone close to them to be the only experience worse than being bullied. Dr. James Dobson recognizes bullying as "a huge, huge problem in this culture." In a daily broadcast aired on October 25, 2001, he commented, "Kids can be cruel. I recently spoke with a strong Christian family whose son had contemplated suicide because he was being made fun of at school. . . . People say, 'It's an overreaction. Everybody goes through that.' Sure they do. Most of us did. And most of us got through it. But most of us are different for having gone through it."

In that same broadcast, Dr. Dobson shared one reason he feels so strongly about bullying:

> For two years in junior high I was really taking it. I remember one day when I was fourteen that was really terrible. I cried all the way home. As usual, my good dad was there, and he sat me down to talk about it. He talked me down from the precipice. That's really important for you to understand. If [a boy or girl] has parents who are involved, when they run into these things you can work your way through them and release the tensions. But many kids don't have that. There's nobody at home and nobody cares, or they care but are too exhausted to be involved. So the tensions grow. They get angrier, and there's a form of rage that develops inside.

Dr. Dobson was blessed to have a dad who was physically present and knew how to listen to and guide his wounded son. The anger and despair of bullied children who don't have this kind of loving guidance can lead to incredible emotional, relational, and spiritual wounding that may overflow into self-destruction or cause the child to lash out. In June 2002, the American Medical Association reported, "Without intervention, bullying can lead to serious academic, social, emotional and legal problems." A 1998 study revealed that 10 percent of students in the United States who drop out of school do so because of repeated bullying. Even more shocking, it's been discovered that most teenage suicides and school shootings are committed by those who have been bullied or feel victimized or persecuted.

Many parents I talk to are surprised to learn that, as in Debbie's case, girls are bullying other girls. Some researchers believe that bullying by girls is more common than bullying by boys, and some even describe bullying among girls as an "epidemic." Rather than using physical means, most girl bullies resort to relational or verbal bullying. They may isolate another girl from their social circle or gossip maliciously about her.

Experts disagree on what causes some children to respond to bullying by engaging in violence or by committing suicide. But there seems to be a link between these responses and violent music, movies, and video games, which often buttress feelings of low self-esteem and even encourage self-destructive behavior. Many such forms of entertainment elevate violence as an appropriate payback for bullying. As parents, we must evaluate if these forms of entertainment are igniting an already bitter fixation—like pouring gasoline on a smoldering fire.

If your child suffers from unexplained fatigue, fear, sleep disturbances, or vague physical ailments that crop up on school days, he or she may be struggling with someone who is a bully. These may be your only clues, because children who are bullied are usually fearful of reporting it—even to their parents.

It's important to remember, however, that bullying doesn't have to produce devastating, long-term harm. Dr. James Dobson offers this encouragement:

The human personality grows through mild adversity, provided it is not crushed in the process. I have enjoyed happiness and fulfillment thus far my entire lifetime, with the exception of two painful years. Those stressful years occurred during my seventh- and eighth-grade days, lasting through ages thirteen and fourteen. [Yet] these two years have contributed more positive features to my adult personality than any other span of which I am aware.

Resource Box   Helpful Hints

Face Bullying Head-on

Bob Smithouser, youth culture adviser at Focus on the Family, offers these tips for parents whose children are being bullied:

- Assure your child that you are on his or her side and you won't take any action without discussing it first. But also make it clear that your intent is to protect your child.
- Realize that your child is not to blame for being bullied, and refuse to believe any lies being told about him or her. The bully is the disturbed one. Remind your children of their value in your and God's sight, and help them understand that no one can make them feel inferior without their permission.
- Pray with and for your child for protection and wise decision making. Pray for the bully to undergo a heart change. Pray about how you should intervene.
- Chronicle tense encounters in writing. Without exaggerating, note what was said or done, where it took place, who witnessed it, and so on. Beyond being therapeutic, this is especially helpful if outside mediators need to enter the picture.
- Investigate the school's anti-bullying policy. Call and talk to the principal or other authority—not to the bully or the bully's parents. Knowing the amount of support one can expect on campus—and where to go for help—can make a child feel less isolated.
- Help your child learn to rely on trusted peers for support. Peers can provide a crucial safety net for vulnerable young people.

UNVEILING ELECTRONIC STRANGERS

We've explored the need to protect our children from hostile strangers outside the home. Now we must turn our attention to protecting our children inside our homes. We want our homes to be safe for our children. This is why we pay attention to home safety, have rules about activities and behaviors, and teach our children to be responsible and respectful.

But there are other risks to our children's health about which we may not be nearly as vigilant. These threats come into our homes as strangers via television and the Internet. Improper use of electronic media is dramatically harming the physical, emotional, relational, and spiritual health of our children. Parents are the key to protecting them from these potentially evil raiders.

Television: Too Influential to Ignore

Television watching is a huge part of everyday life in America. More than 99 percent of U.S. households have at least one television set, and only 13 percent of them report having only one television. More than half of parents report that their children have televisions in their bedrooms. In addition, 42 percent of children ages nine to seventeen have their own cable or satellite television hookups in their bedrooms. I'm positively shocked by these statistics!

Furthermore, the idea of mom or dad watching television with the children is apparently no longer the norm. Many parents allow their children to watch any programs they want. Considering the explicit sex, violence, nudity, and profanity in many programs, this revelation disturbs me. A study of 450 sixth graders who watch cable TV confirmed my concerns: 66 percent of them watched at least one program a month that contained nudity or heavy sexual content.

During the 1950s, 1960s, and 1970s, television shows were, for the most part, entertaining and positive. But today's most popular shows are likely to include blatant sexual promiscuity, profanity, coarse joking, glaring anti-family subplots, extremely graphic violence, and self-indulgent materialism. Now more than ever, discretion in watching television is essential. To allow our children to watch whatever they want whenever they want to watch it is almost like inviting a complete stranger who doesn't share our morals and values to take care of and teach them. When we place our children in front of the television, we're placing them into the hands of complete strangers—actors, producers, scriptwriters—and that's increasingly risky.

Television has altered the way most children in the United States spend their time. Children in previous eras spent time reading, playing games, and exploring the outdoor world. Today's children spend hours each week with eyes glued to television screens and with bottoms firmly planted on living room rugs or sofas. According to literacy professor Kate Moody, they spend more time with TV than they spend talking to parents, playing with peers, attending school, or reading books—usurping family time, play time, and the reading time that could promote language development.

Many children spend more time with television than they do with any other form of entertainment. A recent Media in the Home survey shows the average child in the United States spends about twenty-five hours a week in front of the television set (including the use of a VCR). Contrast this statistic with the American Academy of Pediatrics' recommendation that children watch no more than one to two hours of "quality" television a day and that children under age two not watch television at all.

Although most parents believe that television is the primary pipeline into their homes for negative social messages (and 90 percent believe it's getting worse), fewer than one in four parents (22 percent) say they've seriously considered getting rid of the television, and the majority of parents still believe television can be beneficial. Many parents believe television is fine in moderation if the right shows are watched, but here's the rub: Many parents are addicted to television themselves.

Resource Box   **Helpful Hints**

A Television-Free Home: Is It for You?

For a variety of healthy reasons, some families have chosen to pull the plug on television. They may do it to promote family closeness, to better control what their children are exposed to, or to stimulate their children's dreams and creativity. You may be amazed by the positive changes in television-free homes documented by professor Barbara Brock of Eastern Washington University.

Television-free families showed a high degree of relational health. They were more likely to participate in sit-down dinners, family activities, hobbies, games, chores, pet care, walking, music, gardening, going to movies, sleeping, sports, community service, housecleaning, outdoor activities, and writing. Parents in television-free homes had about an hour of meaningful conversation *every day* with their children (compared to the national average of between five and six minutes a day). Nearly 70 percent of parents felt their children were getting along better with no television.

More than 80 percent of parents in one study believed the lack of television was responsible for improved academic work. More than half of the children in Brock's study received mostly or all A's in school. Television-free children have a longer attention span. As children read more, their grades improve.

Children in television-free homes were more active physically than other children their age. One-fourth of the children studied were physically active thirteen or more hours per week, which paid off in improved physical health. Only 7 percent of television-free children were ten or more pounds overweight, and fewer than two in one hundred had an eating disorder.

It's also interesting that the computer and Internet did not take over television's role in most homes. Although 98 percent of television-free families own a computer, many television-free children actually report being bored with computer or video games.

Contrary to what one might think, children in television-free homes aren't missing out on anything; in fact, as Barbara Brock observes, the vast majority of responses indicate that TV watching families are the ones missing out—missing out, in fact, on life.

What Does Television Really Do to Our Children?

In their book *How to Get the Best Out of TV,* Dale Mason, Karen Mason, and Ken Wales have a fascinating chapter titled "Seven Shocking Reasons to Watch What Kids Watch!" Let me share with you some of the research they've accumulated.

Current research seems to indicate that television viewing today is associated with aggression, a desensitization to violence, and increased fear. Here are a few conclusions drawn from the massive evidence showing that too much television viewing is harming our children's health.

Too Much Television Viewing Can Lower Creativity

Television has been accurately described as a sort of plug-in drug. It can gradually lull viewers, especially children, into noninteractive passivity. Youngsters who should be reading, playing, running, and exploring end up exercising only their eyelids as they sit spellbound in front of the tube. Those who have studied childhood viewing habits often conclude that children who are obsessed by TV are less creative and more passive. Evidence also points to the fact that television interferes with the capacity to entertain oneself and stifles the ability to express ideas logically and sensitively. What's more, as many children pattern their free play after television programs, they no longer envision new situations or new worlds—and imagination is stifled and creativity hampered.

Too Much Television Viewing Can Lead to Physical Health Concerns

There appears to be a strong relationship between the amount of time children spend in front of the television and weight problems. A study of more than a thousand children between the ages of two and twelve revealed this somber finding: Children who watch two to four hours of television a day have a *significantly* higher likelihood of high cholesterol levels (above 200) than those who watch less than two hours a day. Research by preventive medicine specialist Dr. Robert Klesges found that children watching TV tended to burn fewer calories per minute than those engaged in active play. The surprising finding: They tended to burn fewer calories than those who were reading or doing nothing—in fact, almost as few as children who were sleeping. Fortunately, these effects seem to be reversible. Other studies have showed that overweight children lost weight simply by decreasing their television viewing.

Viewing Television Violence Can Shape Our Children's Minds and Hearts

During a child's estimated 22,000 hours in front of television by age fourteen, he or she will have witnessed assaults on more than 18,000 individuals, usually without any negative consequences. A 1995 study funded by the cable television industry tracked 2,500 hours of television programming and reported that 57 percent of television programs contain psychologically harmful violence. Is it any wonder we see children who "play" violently, use foul language, and engage in fights?

Studies by George Gerbner have shown that children who watch a lot of television are more likely to think that the world is a mean and dangerous place. Pennsylvania State University researchers noticed real differences in behavior between preschool children who watched aggressive, violent cartoons and those who watched nonviolent ones. They found that those who watched the violent shows—even if they were just funny cartoons—were more likely to lash out at their playmates, argue, disobey class rules, and leave tasks unfinished than those who watched the nonviolent shows. Even more alarming, the effects of television violence on children are long term! Researcher Leonard

Eron found that children who watched many hours of television violence while in elementary school tended to show a higher level of aggressive behavior when they became teenagers, and they were more likely to be arrested and prosecuted for criminal acts as adults.

Dose of Wisdom

Like the sorcerer of old, the television set casts its magic spell, freezing speech and action, turning the living into silent statues so long as the enchantment lasts. The primary danger of the television lies not so much in the behavior it produces as in the behavior it prevents: the talks, the games, the family festivities and arguments through which character is formed. Turning on the television set can turn off the process that transforms children into people.

Urie Bronfenbrenner, child development expert

Too Much Television Viewing Can Decrease Family Interaction

Tuning in to television causes viewers to tune out those around them. When we parents fail to limit television watching, we waste opportunities for children to learn how to relate to other people. As a family's television time increases, family interaction decreases. Yet, there's a longing in the hearts of most young people today to have a deeper relationship with their families. Three-fourths of the 750 ten- to sixteen-year-olds who participated in a nationwide survey said that if they had a choice between watching TV and spending time with their families, they'd opt for family time.

Children of all ages need loving, caring, *daily* contact with their parents. They seek from their parents both reassurance that they are loved and instruction for navigating adult society. This interaction is as important as food, water, and fresh air, but television can take it away. One deeply hurt teenager told me, "I'm not as important to my mom and dad as their television." This teenager actually *wanted* to get closer to her parents, but their television addiction made an intimate family relationship an all-but-impossible dream.

When your child wants your attention, do you sometimes respond with, "Shhh, I'm watching television"? If you do, it strongly indicates that television is your priority. When we put television ahead of people, it reveals a lot about the value we place on others.

Too Much Television Viewing Can Lower School Performance

Only a few television programs teach important skills such as math, reading, science, and problem solving. The vast majority of programs, including nearly every cartoon show, have virtually no educational value. The more time a child spends watching these types of shows, the poorer his or her overall school performance and the lower his or her standardized test scores.

Many educators criticize television for promoting passive learning and shorter attention spans so that children have difficulty concentrating and working hard to solve problems. In addition, the more time children spend in front of a television, the less time they have available to spend on homework or in stimulating interactions with their parents or other people.

The research convinces me that television can have a devastating impact on our children's health. We parents simply must transform this menacing enemy into a potentially beneficial ally. It's imperative that we control the amount and content of television our children watch. The consequences of not doing so may be catastrophic.

Resource Box   **Helpful Hints**

Tips for Taming Television

Television viewing doesn't have to be out of control. Parents can set limits and teach children to make wise viewing choices. Consider the following suggestions (adapted from a sidebar in Dr. Daphne Miller's WebMD article titled "Television's Effects on Kids: It Can Be Harmful").

- Consider becoming a TV-free home. Short of that, limit television viewing to no more than two hours a day for everyone in the household older than the age of two. It's crucial for parents to stick to this rule, because children imitate their parents' behavior.

- Choose shows with your children, steering them toward educational programs. Avoid violent shows. If you have trouble controlling what your children watch, consider putting a lockbox on the television.

- Have your children pick shows that will not interfere with daily routines such as meals, homework, and bedtime.

- Do not use the television as a baby-sitter; instead, watch shows with your children. This is especially important for children under age ten because they may need your guidance to distinguish between fantasy and reality.

- Avoid snacking or eating family meals while watching television.

- Don't allow your children to have televisions in their bedrooms. It will only make it more difficult for you to regulate what your children watch, and it does nothing to promote family togetherness.

- Most important, encourage your children to do things other than watch television. Do an art project together, read a book, or get out of the house and go to the playground or zoo. In other words, don't watch life. Live it!

The Internet: Its Dark Side

Because you desire to raise highly healthy children, you should be concerned about another electronic stranger in your home, namely, the Internet. It can be a wonderful place to find information and order products and a great way to communicate via email, but it has an extremely dark side. Stalkers, pornographers, thieves, and all manner of evil people lurk in cyberspace, just as in real life. They want to steal your money, corrupt your morals, bend your ethics, or, worse yet, target your children. So you must be aware of how your children use the Internet.

Consider the facts:

- Nearly one in five American youths who surfed the Internet regularly were targets of unwanted sexual attention.
- Pedophiles and child predators are not just dirty old men in raincoats. The FBI has warned that "computer-based sex offenders may be any age or sex."
- Adult sex offenders and rip-off artists often pose as kids in chat rooms, trying to exchange personal information—such as addresses and phone numbers—with children. Exchanging this information puts not only your children at risk but also your entire family and finances.

It's up to us as parents to take an active interest in our children's online activity. If your children use the Internet, you need to develop "Internet parenting expertise." You must regularly ask your children to show you the sites they visit. You have the right and obligation to know who is sending them email. The bottom line is that children are not safe on the Internet, not even for a moment. If you let your children run wild in cyberspace, they will get hurt.

Parenting with Dignity suggests that the best ways to protect your children online are to show them how to use the Internet safely and to ask them to follow some simple rules. Make sure you explain the rules and the reasons behind them. You may even want to post these rules on the computer:

- **Always** use a "screen name." *Never* disclose any details about yourself— your real name, the school you attend, your age, your phone number, or where you live—not even the town or state.
- **Always** tell your parents if you receive any emails or other communications that are frightening or upsetting.
- **Never** exchange photographs over the Internet (or through the mail).
- **Never** agree to meet in person anyone you met in a chat room. Tell your parents immediately if someone offers to meet you.
- **Never** give your password to anyone.
- **Never** enter private chat rooms.
- **Never** accept anything a person says online at face value.

What else can you do? Equip your computer with a filter, such as Cyber Patrol and Net Nanny, so your children cannot wander into inappropriate areas. If your browser includes built-in filters, use them. Also check the major search engines. Many of them have the ability to turn on a child-safe mode. For more about Internet filtering, access the FilterReview.com website or the Parenting with Dignity website (as well as the above filter websites) via my website at www.highlyhealthy.net.

Always monitor your children's computer activities. Place computers used by children in a common room such as the family room or in places that are visible from places you normally occupy. This way you can watch over your children as they work and play on the computer. Monitor the amount of time your children spend on the Internet. Monitor their activities directly by being with them and helping them surf the Web. Monitor their activities indirectly by checking their cookie files, browser caches, history lists, recycle bins, and so on. If you don't know how to do this, ask a friend who has computer experience—or ask a teenager. When Scott was a preteen, he and I agreed to monitor each other's computer time and the Internet sites we visited. (He taught me how to do this.) Not only was I able to check on him, he became my accountability partner to help protect me from the dangers of the Internet.

Most important, talk to your children. Explain the dangers of the Internet. Learn with them what to avoid. Get them to tell you when undesirable things such as pornographic spam or emails appear. As a parent, you *must* be willing to practice healthy Internet habits yourself. When it comes to becoming highly healthy, both children *and* parents need to consider all the potentially harmful effects of an electronic pipeline into your home.

Resource Box   **Helpful Hints**

If your children use the Internet, always be on the lookout for the warning signs of trouble in cyberspace:

- Your child spends long hours online (especially in the evening).
- You receive phone calls from people you don't know.
- Unsolicited gifts arrive via the mail.
- Your child turns off the computer when you enter the room.
- Your child withdraws from family activities.
- Your child is reluctant to discuss Internet activities.

PROTECTING YOUR CHILDREN FROM SUBSTANCE ABUSE

Recently I spoke with a pastor who said something that shocked and disappointed me. He shared about how terrible it was that several teens in his church had developed drug or alcohol addictions. Then he said, "At least we won't have that problem in our family."

"How do you know?" I inquired.

With a baffled look on his face, he responded, "Well, my kids have said this just will not be a problem. I'm sure it won't."

The "I won't have to worry about it" attitude—or delusion—is one of the most dangerous attitudes a parent can have. I commonly saw it in the parents of the substance-abusing children and teens I cared for in my practice. The majority of parents (79 percent), however, do worry about protecting their children from alcohol and drugs, and 55 percent of parents say they worry about it a lot.

Concern about drug and alcohol use is not limited to parents of teens. One national survey showed that parents of five- to nine-year-olds are just as concerned as parents of teens, and it seems their fears are well-founded. One survey of seventh graders showed that 29 percent reported using alcohol at least once in the previous six months!

Resource Box   **Helpful Hints**

Why Kids Use Drugs and Alcohol

Children use alcohol and drugs for a variety of reasons, including the following:

- having fun and gaining peer acceptance, self-confidence, identity, status, security, cultural identification, power, physical performance, peace of mind, the rush of taking risks, heightened sensory experience, or mystical experience
- being curious to find out what it's like
- coping with poverty; school, family, or social problems; emotional or sexual problems; or communication problems
- coping with failure or boredom
- having a lack of knowledge about the effects of alcohol and other drugs, about where to seek help, and about how to say no and defend the choice not to use them
- wanting to be noticed, respected, and accepted—needs that are crucial for a child's emotional well-being; when

these needs aren't being met, children are more likely to take risks to fulfill them. Advertisements, television programs, and films glamorize alcohol and drug use as the way to meet these needs.

None of us want to believe that our children are vulnerable to substance abuse, but the reality is they are. A recent ad campaign labels parents as "the anti-drug," but I've found that most parents don't know how to discuss the topic with their children. Many parents believe they lack knowledge about the topic or think they'll have no impact on their children. Yet studies clearly reveal that parents can have an amazing impact in protecting their children from substance abuse. The two keys are (1) that they *strongly disapprove* of substance abuse (including parents themselves not abusing drugs, alcohol, or tobacco) and (2) that they *lovingly communicate* this disapproval to their children.

Our children observe and learn from the ways in which we behave. They watch what we do with much more attention than they listen to what we say. They are designed to imitate us, follow us, and try to be like us—for good or for bad. That's why my son, Scott, used to put on my robe and loafers, and why my daughter, Kate, used to put on Barb's makeup. They were trying on adult roles to see what fit.

So take a good look at your use of medical and nonmedical drugs. Your actions in this area exert a powerful influence on your child—even when he or she is very young. Ask yourself, *Am I showing my child the behaviors I want him or her to copy? If not, how can I change my drug-using behavior?*

In addition to being aware of what you're modeling for your children, you can take positive steps to decrease their chances of experimenting with or abusing substances:

- First, prepare yourself to talk with your children, at an age-appropriate level, about drug use. It's never too early to start a dialogue. A young child can benefit from discussions about medicine and why it should never be taken without a parent's permission and supervision. An older child may want to know more specifically about cigarettes, alcohol, and illicit drugs. (Many experts say the best age to begin educating children about alcohol and other drugs is between six and nine years of age.) A teenager may be mainly curious about illicit drugs. Get the most up-to-date information about drugs and talk about it with your children. You don't have to be an expert, but you do need to be knowledgeable.

- Second, set clear, reasonable limits. Let your children know that under no circumstances are they to experiment with drugs. Explain why this behavior is unacceptable and what the consequences will be for not meeting this expectation. (Some drugs, for example, are highly addictive with only one use!) Remember, children behave more responsibly when parents set limits. Check your disciplinary style. Do you provide discipline that is firm and consistent, but not unfair or overbearing? Children who abuse substances often come from families where the discipline is either extremely restrictive or permissive.

- Third, resist the urge to lecture, and be prepared to listen. Keep communication lines open. Your children should feel that they can approach you for advice about even the most difficult issues. While you may hear things you'd rather not hear, at least your children are asking you instead of an unknown and possibly unreliable source. Playing together, working together, and sharing interesting and exciting experiences as a family can develop mutual caring and respect within a family. Private time alone with each child is also important in encouraging communication and sharing of confidences. A strong and loving parent-child relationship can give both children and parents the firm foundation to withstand difficult situations.

- Fourth, don't be afraid to ask other people for advice. A child doesn't arrive with an instruction manual. Asking for help when you're at a loss is a mark of excellent parenting, not a sign of failure.

In spite of your best efforts, your children may still abuse alcohol or drugs. Remember, however, that the choice is theirs, not yours. Even if you're convinced that your children will never use alcohol or drugs, it's wise to be aware of signs of substance abuse. You don't want to be the last person to know, and you do want to become aware of alcohol or drug use in its early stages when effective intervention is easier.

Signs of Alcohol or Drug Use

Occasional alcohol or drug use is difficult to detect. Some young people may have only a few symptoms, and some will have none. Many symptoms can be present for reasons other than alcohol or drug involvement. However, telltale signs that may point to alcohol or drug use include the following:

- drug paraphernalia or drugs (including pacifiers) in the house
- decreased or altered liquor supplies in the house
- family members' prescription drugs are disappearing
- burn marks on fingers or bruised inner arms
- reddened eyes
- loss of appetite, craving for sweets, weight loss
- sleep disturbance
- inexplicable mood changes—euphoria followed by tenseness and edginess
- estrangement from family
- new friends, strange phone calls, secretiveness
- drop in school performance—not necessarily from A's to D's, but from A's to B's and C's
- caring less about school, sports, hobbies
- money or other valuables come up missing
- vague weekend "party" plans

After a recent Thanksgiving meal, our family was talking and laughing together. Scott, a college student at the time, looked at me and then his mom and said, "Mom and Dad, I'm thankful for you. I'm thankful you were my parents. And I'm thankful for the home you provided for us."

Kate nodded her head, "I'm thankful, too. I'm thankful for all you did to keep us safe—to protect us and provide for us."

It was an extremely emotional moment for Barb and me. We were so thankful for the gift that our two children are to us. We were thankful to have been taught that providing protection for our children was one of our most important jobs as their parents. Adequate protection laid the foundation for Barb and me to work on nurturing deep and meaningful family relationships—and that's the essential we will explore in the next chapter.

Chapter Seven

Nurture Family Relationships

Barb and I met when we were in kindergarten. Our families were friends, so as we grew up, we enjoyed good times together and shared many similar experiences. Our dads, for example, taught at a college and made family a priority. We each had three siblings and professional moms who set aside their careers when we were younger to pour out love on us and devote energy to raising us. Our parents practiced strict discipline and had high expectations for us. We were required to eat breakfast and supper with the family. We took vacations and developed family holiday traditions. Not only were our parents committed to us, but our extended families as well—aunts, uncles, cousins, and grandparents—encouraged, nurtured, admonished, supported, loved, and protected us.

We truly were blessed to have been raised in nurturing families and to have parents who were committed to each other for life. The word *divorce* wasn't in their vocabulary. No matter what trouble or difficulty might be experienced, staying together as a family was a high priority. These commitments to family and marriage provided a strong model and foundation for Barb and me. As our college careers came to an end and I asked Barb to marry me, we looked forward to living close to our families and raising a large family.

Yet, societal views of marriage and family were changing at the time we got married. Families, as Barb and I had known them, were becoming more uncommon. Not everyone was convinced that marriage was nurturing or healthy—or even right.

In his 1970 book *Future Shock,* Alvin Toffler claimed that the family would lose the ability to convey its values to following generations. He predicted that temporary marriages would become widely accepted and recommended that young adults enter into trial marriages, which he called "recognized pre-marriage." About the same time, British psychotherapist David Cooper authored *The Death of the Family* and recommended that society abolish traditional marriage and family in favor of new forms of human relationships. And Shirley MacLaine, actress and self-appointed spiritual guru, made this comment back in 1971: "I don't think it's desirable to conform to having one mate, and for those two people to raise children. But everyone believes that's the ideal. They go around frustrated most of their lives because they can't find one mate. . . . To whom does monogamy make sense?" Many others joined these "family experts" in predicting that marriage, as the basis of nurturing family relationships, was unnecessary and doomed to disappear.

What has happened since their pronouncements? The 2000 U.S. Census Bureau Report has confirmed that the institution of marriage is unraveling. The facts speak for themselves:

- With a divorce rate of more than 50 percent, more than a million children experience their parents' divorce each year.
- In 2000, for the first time in our nation's history, traditional nuclear families dropped below 25 percent of households.
- Thirty-three percent of all babies were born to unmarried women, compared to only 3.8 percent in 1940. In the African-American community, nearly 70 percent of babies were born to single moms.
- About half of the children in our country spend at least part of their childhood in single-parent, grandparent, foster-parent, or cohabiting-parent homes.
- More than 3.3 million children lived with an unmarried parent and the parent's cohabiting partner. Cohabitation now impacts three children for every one child impacted by divorce.

FAMILY HEALTH AFFECTS CHILDREN'S HEALTH

We simply cannot deny that these trends have a negative impact on children. Distinguished Rutgers sociologist David Popenoe makes this observation:

If the family trends of recent decades are extended into the future, the result will not only be growing uncertainty within marriage, but the gradual elimination of marriage in favor of casual liaisons oriented to adult expressiveness and self-fulfillment. The problem with this scenario is that children will be harmed.

I wholeheartedly agree. An ever-increasing number of children have several "moms" or "dads," perhaps six or eight "grandparents," and dozens of half siblings. Little girls and boys are trundled through an ever-changing array of living arrangements, houses, and communities. Social historian Barbara Dafoe Whitehead describes the stresses children experience when their families fall apart:

> All this uncertainty can be devastating to children. Anyone who knows children knows that they are deeply conservative creatures. They like things to stay the same. . . . Children are particularly set in their ways when it comes to family, friends, neighborhoods, and schools. Yet when a family breaks up, all these things may change.

The link between the health of a family and the health of its children is undeniable. Scientific research now shows that the demise of traditional marriages, which I define as the lifelong legal, physical, emotional, social, and spiritual union of one man and one woman, is devastating to our children's health. Parental divorce is estimated to increase children's risk of developing health problems by 50 percent. Although no family is perfect, children of divorced, never-married, blended, same-sex, or cohabiting parents face higher health risks and are likely to suffer emotionally, academically, and economically. When researchers look at virtually every measure of child well-being, they find that children born to or adopted by first-time married partners do significantly better in *all* measures of health than children in any other family category.

So if we want our children to be as healthy as possible, we must take into account the connection between family health and children's health. Family relationships are important. God designed them to be that way. We need to recognize the risks children face when their family relationships are broken and shattered. We all need to learn the steps we can take to repair the damage of broken family relationships and thereby improve the health of our families and children. But before we learn these steps, we must honestly face what we're up against. Let me briefly highlight the evidence showing how the health of the family affects a child's well-being.

Impact of Family Health on Education

Scientists at the Child Study Center at the University of Ottawa found that 30 percent of the children in their study whose parents divorced "experienced a marked decrease in their academic performance." According to another study, children from divorced homes are 70 percent more likely to have been expelled or suspended from school than those living with biological parents. Children living with never-married mothers are twice as likely to be expelled or suspended.

A study published in 2002, which reviewed more than one hundred studies published over the preceding twenty years, found that children living without their natural fathers were three times as likely to have difficulty getting along with other people and to struggle at school. As teenagers, they were twice as likely to drink, smoke, take drugs, play truant, and leave high school without graduating. As adults, children from broken homes are twice as likely to have no academic degree and to be unemployed.

Impact of Family Health on Physical Health

Children from broken homes are fifty percent more likely to suffer health problems and five times more likely to suffer abuse. Those who live with never-married mothers have an increased risk of speech defects. Children living with formerly married mothers and those living with mother and stepfather are at increased risk of frequent headaches, and those who live with formerly married mothers have a 50 percent greater risk of having asthma.

Babies born to single mothers are more likely to be born into poverty and have low birth weights, making them susceptible to respiratory distress syndrome, hypoglycemia, jaundice, and other metabolic and neurological maladies. They are also less likely to be fully immunized and are 2.4 times more likely to die of sudden infant death syndrome than babies born to married mothers.

Impact of Family Health on Psychological Health

Children from single-parent families experience more psychological and emotional problems than children living with both parents. Nearly 20 percent of children living with only their biological mother exhibit significant emotional or behavioral problems, compared to only 8 percent of children living with both parents.

Child psychologist Judith Wallerstein, who has conducted extensive studies on the psychological impact of divorce on children, found that children of divorce often experience feelings of rejection, loneliness, anger, guilt, anxiety, and fear of abandonment, as well as a deep, persistent yearning for the absent parent. Five years after the divorce, 37 percent of the children she studied were moderately or severely depressed. These emotional and behavioral effects often last through the teen years and into adulthood, a finding confirmed by a thirty-three-year study that showed children of divorce to be more than twice as likely to be afflicted with emotional problems, such as depression or anxiety, well into their twenties or early thirties.

Impact of Family Health on Social Behavior

Several studies show that children of divorce are far more likely to be delinquent, commit crimes, engage in premarital sex, and bear children out of wedlock during adolescence and young adulthood. As adults, children of broken homes are three times as likely to be caught offending and go to jail. Teenagers living without their natural fathers are twice as likely to drink, smoke, and take drugs. The psychological damage inflicted on children during and after divorce seems to be responsible for their greater propensity toward unhappiness and self-destructive behavior.

Seldom does social science reach as solid a conclusion as it has on the evidence that strong families and marriages are essential to the well-being of children. Research from the world's leading academic institutions shows that when marriages are strong, adults, children, and society will be strong. There is no better place to nurture highly healthy children than in a home with a happily married mom and dad.

Dose of Wisdom

Despite the loud voices criticizing marriage and the family, most parents realize how important the traditional two-parent family is to raising highly healthy children. A worldwide survey revealed that support for the traditional family is strongly rooted among diverse cultures around the globe. Not only are people significantly concerned about family-related issues, but a surprisingly large percent agree on what constitutes a family. Eighty-six percent of respondents outside the United States said that children should be raised by a mother and father who are married to each other!

Dr. Walt Larimore

WHAT MAKES A FAMILY HEALTHY?

Critics of traditional marriage and family frequently argue that it isn't the formal structure but the *quality* of family relationships that matters. Psychologists Louise Silverstein and Carl Auerbach, for example, believe it isn't marriage but "the stability of the emotional connection and the predictability of the caretaking relationship [that] are the significant variables that predict positive child adjustment." I agree that the quality of family relationships *does* make a huge difference, and stability and predictability *are* essential in the life of a highly healthy child. But the research and thousands of years of human history show that stability and predictability are most likely to occur in a married, two-parent (a mom and a dad) family. This family structure is best equipped to provide children with the parental love, guidance, and resources they need in order to become highly healthy adults.

Let me share an example of the incredible comfort and security the lifelong commitment Barb and I made to each other provided our children. One night at bedtime, when Kate was only five or six years old, she asked, "Daddy?"

"Yes, pumpkin."

"Will you ever leave us?"

"You mean to go out of town?" I asked.

She thought for a minute, and then her eyes filled with tears. "No, Daddy. Will you ever leave us like Janie's daddy left her?"

I smiled and wiped a tear that was falling down her cheek. "Honey, I'm committed to your mom, to you, and to Scott for life. I promised my parents and your mommy's parents that I would love your mommy for life. Even more important, I promised God I would love your mom and you for life."

Now it was Kate's turn to smile. She took a deep breath and exhaled, as though the burdens of the world had just been lifted off her shoulders. Maybe they had been.

In real life, one cannot separate the many contributions of a married father and mother. Much of what each parent contributes to a child is unique and irreplaceable. I think of several examples from my own childhood. I remember my dad coming home from work and hugging my mom. When I got home from school each day, my mom and I would sit down and chat about my day before I'd run out the door to play. I remember Dad taking me to church on Ash Wednesday. I was only in elementary school at the time, but afterward we'd go to Bob Price's Rexall drugstore to sit at the grill and have biscuits and coffee—just like "real men"!

My parents, of course, were nowhere near perfect. They never took a parenting class. They grew up during the Great Depression and weren't highly expressive with their love or emotion. They were *very* strict disciplinarians. Yet, looking back on my childhood and comparing it with what research has documented and with what the ancient wisdom of Scripture tells us, my parents truly fulfilled their unique God-given roles. Together they provided a healthy foundation—the family stability and caring relationships—for their children.

Popular statements that family processes are more important than family structure usually fail to recognize the truth that the mother's and father's roles in nurturing a family are neither independent nor dispensable. Each parent's role complements the other. Each parent excels at certain jobs. Neither can fulfill the role of the other.

The social science research confirms both that dads are not moms and that dads are as essential as moms. A father can help a child learn to separate from the mom when that time comes; a mom cannot. A father usually supports a child's adventure-seeking behavior; moms usually do not. Dads are often better than moms at helping children learn to master frustration. They also tend to stretch their children's communication skills in preparation for worldly dialogue. Having a mother and a father helps a child learn to form relationships with both sexes and allows a child to observe a heterosexual relationship in action. Let's briefly consider the unique roles of a dad and a mom.

The Dad's Role

Although fatherlessness is epidemic in America, with 34 percent of all children living apart from their biological fathers, children need their dads. An analysis of nearly a hundred studies on parent-child relationships by the National Fatherhood Initiative reveals that father love is as important as mother love in predicting the social, emotional, and cognitive development and functioning of children and young adults. Another group of researchers, looking at the same studies, found that a loving and nurturing father was as important for a child's happiness, well-being, and social and academic success as a loving and nurturing mother. Furthermore, some studies show father love to be a better predictor than mother love (and sometimes the sole significant predictor) for certain outcomes, including delinquency and conduct problems, substance abuse, and overall mental health and well-being.

Fathers who live with their children are more likely to have close, enduring relationships with their children than those who do not. In fact, the best predictor of father presence is marital status. Compared to children born within marriage, children born to cohabiting parents are three times as likely to experience father absence, and children born to unmarried, noncohabiting parents are four times as likely to live in a father-absent home. About 40 percent of children in father-absent homes have not seen their father during the past year, and 50 percent of children living apart from their father have never set foot in their father's home.

The results of these statistics in the daily lives of children are truly tragic. I saw the dreadful effects virtually every day in my practice, as do teachers, school administrators, and police officers. One principal told me, "Walt, give me fifteen to twenty minutes with a child, especially a boy, and I can tell you if he's fatherless or not. I can predict it accurately more than 98 percent of the time."

Studies show that children who don't live with their biological fathers are at least two to three times more likely to be poor; to use drugs; to experience educational, health, emotional, and behavioral problems; to be victims of child abuse; and to engage in criminal behavior than their peers who live with their married parents. In contrast, children with involved, loving fathers are significantly more likely to do well in school, have healthy self-esteem, exhibit empathy and pro-social behavior, and avoid high-risk behaviors such as drug use, truancy, and criminal activity. The closeness a child feels to his or her dad is one of the best predictors of positive outcomes. Even an uninvolved father, if present, is significantly better than no father.

Dose of Wisdom

If our society cares about its children, we must recognize the importance of married fatherhood. And, even more important, we must reduce the high levels of fatherlessness that bode ill for our children and our nation's future.

Wade F. Horn, clinical child psychologist

However, fatherlessness does not condemn any particular child to the social problems of educational failure, drug addiction, or a life of crime. Marriage, by itself, does not guarantee good parenting or highly healthy children. In fact, many children from single-parent families and blended families are healthy. Their well-being is almost always due to the herculean efforts of the single mother or the blended parents. There are great stepfathers who love and care for their stepchildren in remarkably effective ways. To ignore or demean these incredible efforts undertaken by loving and caring single and blended parents and stepparents is not only insulting but evil.

On the other hand, to argue that fatherhood is not essential because some healthy children grow up without an involved father is a weak argument. It's like saying smoking isn't dangerous because it may not kill some who smoke. The truth is, smoking harms many, if not most smokers. In the same way, while growing up fatherless may not irretrievably harm all children who live without a father, it does make them less likely to be highly healthy.

Resource Box   *Helpful Hints*

Looking for some provocative tips on how to become a better father? Look at the Internet-based, hour-long course on "10 Ways to Be a Better Dad." Complete with video clips and notes, this free class may be just what you need to improve your fathering skills. You can find it at my website (www.highlyhealthy.net).

The Mom's Role

The relationship between a mother and her child is as unique and important as that between a father and his child. Children respond to their moms and dads differently. We saw this so vividly with our son, Scott. At times he responded best to Barb; at other times he needed time with me. I could never have given Scott the things that only Barb was designed to give him. In our family, I was the sterner disciplinarian—the one who represented justice more than grace. Barb's feminine touch and intuition could read Scott and his emotions much more quickly than I, however. As his mom, she was the vessel of mercy and grace.

Much research confirms the overwhelming value of a mother's nurture, love, and support. The responsibilities and rewards of motherhood cannot be successfully delegated. Nannies, au pairs, baby-sitters, and relatives may be necessary, but they can never be mom. Developmental psychologist Brenda

Hunter believes there's no substitute not only for mom, but for mom being at home with her young children. Her investigation leads her to conclude that a mother plays a powerful role in a child's development, particularly her unique contribution to the formation of conscience and empathy.

Numerous studies show that one of the best ways to build strong independence in children is for their mothers to meet their needs when the children are very young. These children are more likely to make wise, independent decisions and not just run with the crowd. In addition, they are less likely to be abnormally dependent on others or to become codependent adults or spouses. In fact, Jay Belsky, professor of human development at Pennsylvania State University, warns that "extensive nonmaternal care in the first year is a risk factor in the development of insecure infant-parent attachment relationships." Nationally renowned pediatrician T. Berry Brazelton and child psychiatrist Stanley Greenspan insist, "In the first three years, every child needs one or two primary caregivers who remain in a steady, intimate relationship with that child." They specify two activities in which young children need to spend at least two-thirds of their waking time: (1) interactions with the environment that are facilitated by their caregiver, and (2) direct interaction with the caregiver—cuddling, holding, shared pretend play, and funny face games, for example. They also recommend that mothers be available enough so they or the children don't have to be measuring each moment of time. Because this type of care isn't typically available in day care, Brazelton and Greenspan don't recommend full-time day care for infants and toddlers *if* the parents are able to provide high-quality care themselves and *if* the parents have reasonable options.

Dose of Wisdom

A mother's job is making memories. Whether we spend long hours reading to our children or creating savory meals, we are contributing to the concept our children will have of home. We are stockpiling memories for them to use in the years ahead. We are filling the corners of their minds with sights and sounds and smells that will reemerge just when they need to remember that somewhere they are loved, whether they falter or whether they flourish.

Linda Burton, cofounder, Family and Home Network

As essential as the mother-child relationship is during early childhood, it doesn't end when a child starts school or leaves the primary grades behind. Moms continue to be a major influence on their children's health throughout adolescence. An old Spanish proverb says, "An ounce of mother is worth a pound of priest," and current research on teens and their risk of drug abuse supports this observation:

- 71 percent of teens report having an excellent or very good relationship with mom; only 58 percent have such a relationship with dad.
- More than twice as many teens say it's easier to talk to mom than dad about drugs (57 percent versus 26 percent).
- Twice as many teens who never used marijuana credit mom as credit dad with this decision (29 percent versus 13 percent).
- Teens are three times more likely to rely solely on mom than solely on dad when they have important decisions to make (27 percent versus 9 percent).

What about Same-Sex-Partner Families?

A growing number of voices are claiming that homosexual couples can provide healthy homes for children. Many are pushing for the legalization of adoption, foster parenting, and coparenting by same-sex couples. Sympathetic pediatricians formulated an endorsement of homosexual parenting that was approved in February 2002 by the American Academy of Pediatrics (AAP). Most of the news stories about the AAP statement failed to reveal how controversial this recommendation is or how limited the research is on which the endorsement was based.

Most of the research cited by the AAP, however, doesn't support their claims. For example, an article in the *American Sociological Review* (by authors who "oppose discrimination on the basis of sexual orientation") reviewed twenty-one studies of homosexual parenting and acknowledged that "researchers frequently downplay findings indicating difference" in outcomes for children of gay and straight parents. Various studies of lesbian mothers (the most frequent homosexual parenting model) found that their children are less likely to conform to traditional gender roles and more likely to engage in homosexual experimentation. In addition, their daughters are reported to be more sexually adventurous and less chaste. The *American Sociological Review* study also found that 64 percent of young adults raised by lesbian mothers reported considering having same-sex relationships, compared to only 17 percent of young adults in heterosexual families.

Research on homosexuals has shown that they are more promiscuous than heterosexuals; that even their long-term relationships are characterized by less faithfulness and less stability; and that they have higher rates of sexually transmitted disease, substance abuse, mental health problems, and domestic violence. Furthermore, lesbian coparent relationships are more likely to break up than heterosexual marriages. None of these documented outcomes are healthy for children.

These outcomes and the strong tendency among children of same-sex partners to consider same-sex relationships for themselves are of great concern. No serious scientists believe that homosexuality is genetic. There is a growing recognition among some psychologists that homosexuality is related to family dysfunction and issues occurring during the development of the child, and therefore may be preventable. Based on current research on same-sex parenting and a new understanding about the development of homosexuality, it is highly unlikely that same-sex-partner families are, in general, healthy for children.

EVERY FAMILY CAN BECOME MORE HEALTHY

I hope by now it's fairly clear that children raised by a mom and dad who are married and committed to each other and their children are more likely to be highly healthy than other children. I suspect that you desire your family to become more highly healthy, but I also suspect that your family, like my family, isn't perfect. In fact, many families—married, two-parent families among them—are unhealthy.

The good news is, no matter how healthy or unhealthy your family is today, you can take steps to improve your family's health. You see, there never has been a perfect family. Broken relationships that impair the health of children have plagued families since Adam and Eve. Imperfect relationships exist in all families, but they tend to be more common and troublesome in dysfunctional families, single-parent families, and blended families. Each of these situations presents both similar and unique health risks to children. In each situation, we parents can take positive steps to improve our family health and lessen the risks to our children.

Healthy Steps for Dysfunctional Families

All families go through times when functioning is impaired by stressful circumstances such as a death in the family, the serious illness of a family member, or the absence of one parent for a long period of time. Healthy families tend to return to normal functioning after the crisis passes. In dysfunctional families, however, the stresses and problems tend to become chronic. The family becomes increasingly unhealthy because of the negative patterns of parental behavior that tend to dominate family life. As a result, children's basic needs aren't being consistently met.

Healthy families may experience episodes of occasional yelling, bickering, misunderstandings, tension, hurt, and anger—just as in dysfunctional families—but these things haven't become a way of life. In healthy families, emotional expression is allowed and accepted. Family members can freely ask for and give attention. Rules tend to remain consistent but are administered with flexibility to adapt to individual needs and situations. Healthy families allow for individuality; each member is encouraged to pursue his or her own interests, and boundaries are honored. In healthy families, children are treated with unconditional respect and love. They don't live in fear of emotional, verbal, physical, spiritual, or sexual abuse. Parents can be counted on to care for their children. Children have appropriate responsibilities and are not expected to take on parental responsibilities. Mistakes are allowed.

In highly unhealthy or dysfunctional families, some or most of these behaviors and practices do not occur. Some parents take a minimalist approach when it comes to caring for their children, leaving them to fend for themselves. Other parents are too heavy-handed, never allowing their children to grow up. Still others are inconsistent or even violate the basic boundaries of appropriate behavior. Each type of dysfunctional family has its own problems, and the unhealthy outcomes vary widely from child to child.

Despite their uniqueness, most dysfunctional families have at least one thing in common: One or both parents grew up in a dysfunctional family. The negative effects of growing up in a dysfunctional family often spill over from one generation to the next. The survival skills that were helpful to the children as they grew up usually go on to cause problems when those children marry and have children of their own. And the Bible indicates that family dysfunction extends not just to the children but to the third and fourth generations. However, there's good news as well. This horrifying cycle *can* be broken.

Getting help from a pastoral or mental health professional is one key strategy for overcoming family dysfunction. Since most children in dysfunctional families have spent years learning and practicing their survival skills, it usually takes a lot of work to learn and practice new skills and behaviors. Yet parents need to take steps to break the cycle and make positive changes in the family so that their children can move down the road toward becoming highly healthy. In addition, support from other healthy adults or family members can help prevent or minimize negative effects. As you read on, several of the suggested steps for single-parent and blended families can also help improve the health of dysfunctional families.

Resource Box   Helpful Hints

Therapy groups—such as Survivors of Incest Anonymous (SIA) and Adult Children of Dysfunctional Families (ACODF)—and self-help groups—such as Adult Children of Alcoholics (ACOA), Al-Anon, and Codependents Anonymous (CoDA)—have many resources and can help dysfunctional families begin to break the cycle of multi-generational dysfunction. You can learn more about these groups at www.highlyhealthy.net.

Healthy Steps for Single-Parent Families

Being a single parent is one of the hardest jobs in the world. Single parents face tremendous pressures in their daily race against the clock. The personal, financial, and time pressures make it extremely difficult to create a healthy family environment in which to raise children. The task can seem overwhelming when single parents recognize and seek to counteract the serious health risks their children face:

- *Child abuse.* The rate of child abuse in single-parent families is nearly twice the rate in two-parent households.
- *Crime.* After adjusting for family background variables such as mothers' education level, race, family income, and number of siblings, as well as neighborhood variables such as unemployment rates and median income, boys who grew up outside of intact marriages were, on average, more than twice as likely as other boys to end up in jail.

- *Drug and alcohol use.* After adjusting for the effects of gender, age, race-ethnicity, family income, and residential mobility, teens in single-parent (and stepparent) families were twice as likely to use illegal drugs compared to teens in intact, two-parent married families.
- *Education.* Even after adjusting for differences in income, children who were born out of wedlock and either remained in single-parent families or whose mothers subsequently married had significantly poorer math and reading scores and lower levels of academic performance than children from continuously married households.
- *Poverty.* Single-parent families are five times as likely to be poor as married-couple families. In 1999, 4.9 percent of married-couple families were living in poverty, compared to 13.6 percent of male householder families with no spouse present and 26.5 percent of female householder families with no spouse present.

The task of financially supporting and raising healthy children by oneself becomes so demanding that single parents often end up becoming depressed or experiencing a myriad of other relational, emotional, or physical health concerns. Those caught in the burden of single parenting need help. They need hope, and they need encouragement. Sadly, some of them turn to cohabitation as a solution.

What about Cohabitation?

I've surprised some of my patients when I vigorously discouraged them from taking this path. The facts about cohabitation are absolutely shocking. Cohabiting couples have nearly none of the physical, emotional, social, and spiritual benefits that married couples enjoy. Furthermore, premarital cohabitation increases the likelihood of divorce by 50 to 80 percent compared to couples who don't cohabit prior to marriage. Cohabiting couples with children number 1.7 million, according to the United States 2000 census, so the impact on children is tremendous.

An enormous body of research shows that children are far better off growing up with single parents than with mothers who live with unrelated males. Compared with married couples or single moms, cohabiting women are more likely to have problems with drugs, alcohol, depression, and sexual faithfulness, as well as with violence and other conflict in the home. The single-parent mom or her children are far more likely to be beaten or sexually abused by a cohabiting male.

Cohabitators experience two to five times more violence than married couples. One 1996 study concluded that living with a stepparent or boyfriend "has turned out to be the most powerful predictor of severe child abuse yet."

Strategies for Single Parents

There are many strategies single parents can use in the task of raising highly healthy children, but cohabitation is not one of them! So where can they go to find relief for their physical, emotional, relational, and spiritual needs? What can they do to compensate for not having a spouse? Thankfully there are antidotes that can make a significant, positive impact—in their lives and in the lives of their children. While the following suggestions can't cure the problem, they can provide some much-needed relief, which can then lead to healthier families and healthier children.

- *Build relationships outside your immediate family.* Single parents should consider how to involve their children in appropriate other-gender mentoring relationships and role models. A great place to look for support is in the extended family. Uncles, cousins, and grandfathers all play vital roles in the developmental process of boys living with a single mom. Outside of the family, church programs, YMCA programs, and camps can offer safe, positive role models for children of all ages.
- *Seek support from your extended family.* Even if they don't live nearby, family members can—and should—pitch in by offering financial assistance. They should offer to host the children for long weekends or during summer vacations. Regular phone calls can provide emotional comfort when life seems overwhelming. A warm, friendly voice speaking a message of love and acceptance is a valuable gift indeed.
- *Find like-minded friends and develop resources.* Since single parents face a difficult uphill battle, they must make connections with like-minded friends and neighbors who can provide support and strength. Socialization is crucial to experiencing high levels of health for any person, and the single parent is no exception. Many single parents find support through jobs, community recreational events, a faith community, support groups, single-parent publications, Internet sites, and so forth. A number of different organizations and ministries (Crown Financial Ministries, for example, which offers free financial advice and materials) can be invaluable resources. You can find out more about Crown Financial Ministries at my website (www.highlyhealthy.net).

- *Connect with a local faith community.* I strongly believe faith communities must become places where single parents can hear a message of grace and acceptance and find help in times of need. In Christianity, the divinely instituted church is to be a family for the familyless. The Bible emphasizes that the local church is obligated to care for widows and orphans: "Religion that God our Father accepts as pure and faultless is this: to look after orphans and widows in their distress." No institution can—and should—care for its widows and orphans better than the church, and a single parent whose spouse no longer lives in the home is indeed a "widow"; the single parent with no extended family in the community is, to my way of thinking, an "orphan."

  A healthy faith community can provide the firm foundation many single parents need: those who can be other-gender role models for the children; those who can provide godly counsel; those who can share Bible studies targeted toward their needs; peers who can offer support and understanding through gifts of time and money; and those who can offer financial support, perhaps by helping the parent set up a home business so she or he can make money at home while caring for young children. Wise, mature members of the faith community can also act as sounding boards for single parents who seek answers to tough questions.

The story for single parents doesn't have to be one of doom and despair. Single moms and dads can find needed support through extended family, the community, and supportive organizations. Yet, it is the faith community—more than any other group—that has the golden opportunity (and obligation) to reach out and support in practical ways those who navigate the deep waters of single parenthood.

Resource Box   *Helpful Hints*

For Internet-active single parents, Focus on the Family hosts a website for single parents. You can access it at www.highlyhealthy.net. Pastor and speaker Gary Richmond has written a wonderful book titled *Successful Single Parenting: Bringing Out the Best in Your Kids.*

Healthy Steps for Blended Families

The vision of the blended family portrayed in the television show *The Brady Bunch* is a myth. The notion that a mom and dad with six children can create one big, happy family without some conflict or rivalries is dramatically unrealistic. It just doesn't happen that way.

Blended families face unique and unsettling challenges that almost always result in significant disillusionment within the first six months of their formation. Although some blended families eventually adjust to their new circumstances, difficulties are frequent and can be severe. The astonishing fact is, most blended families don't make it. The remarriage divorce rate is at least 60 percent.

It is common within a blended family for one or more children to view the new stepparent as a usurper. A child's loyalty to the memory of the departed mother or father is usually intense, so to welcome a newcomer with open arms would be an act of betrayal. This emotional disruption in the child places the stepparent or stepparent-to-be in an impossible bind. What's more, it can affect the child's emotional and relational health in very dysfunctional ways. For example, one child may try to move into the position left by the departed parent and assume the role of a surrogate spouse. These children then attempt to relate to the stepparent as a peer or, even worse, a rival, which isn't healthy for the child or the parent.

Parents considering remarriage should carefully assess their children's feelings and encourage open communication. Potential stepparents should avoid the temptation to "buy" the love of a child. A better way to show love to a potential stepchild is by treating his or her parent with affection and respect.

A more serious problem can develop in the way newly married parents relate to their children. Each stepparent is naturally more committed to his or her own flesh and blood than they are to the children of their new spouse. When fights or insults occur between the two sets of children, a stepparent will almost always be partial to his or her children. Thus the tendency is not to merge like a Brady Bunch but to dissolve into armed camps! When children sense this tension, they almost invariably exploit it to gain power or influence over their siblings—especially their stepsiblings. There's no question that such a scenario is highly *un*healthy emotionally, relationally, and even spiritually.

Dose of Wisdom

First and foremost, the church must convey a message of grace and acceptance [to stepfamilies]. Shaming stepparents for former divorces often burdens stepfamilies. They desperately need to know that they are not second-class when it comes to God's grace. Second, churches must educate remarried couples and stepfamilies in building a successful home. We have to speak to their unique pressures in order to equip them for the challenges ahead. Our pre-remarital counseling must be different in order to educate couples on the road ahead so they can make informed decisions about marriage.

Ron Deal, family life minister; marriage and family therapist

These are only a few of the land mines that threaten blended families. There are many, many others, including managing unrealistic expectations; facing the challenges of blending houses, schools, and friends; dealing with the complexities of financial management; and parenting children who are confused, sad, or even angry about the changing relationships in their lives. Blended family expert Ron Deal believes the single greatest challenge blended couples face is their relationship:

> Marriage is meant to be the foundation to a healthy home; yet in step-families, the couple's relationship is the weakest, least bonded relationship. . . . When stress hits a stepfamily, people tend to divide along biological lines, leaving the couple divided. This is a prescription for trouble. Couples have to make their relationship a high priority or the stepfamily will flounder.

Nevertheless, it is possible to blend families successfully, and many have done it by integrating strategies for building unity in the midst of potentially troublesome blended family dynamics. Together, parents of blended families must establish equitable boundaries for all members of the household and develop traditions to help the two families become a single unit.

It's a difficult task, and it will take time—usually five to seven years. I've always urged parents who are considering this option to seek professional and pastoral counseling as early as possible. Counseling has a cost, but experiencing another broken marriage is even more costly. Let me share Debbie and Scott's story with you.

Debbie and Scott met at church, began dating, fell in love, and planned to marry. Each was a single parent with children at home. They came to me for a premarital evaluation. Physically they were fine, but I knew there were emotional, relational, and spiritual land mines that lay before them. We discussed these, and I gave them resources to read and recommended they seek counseling as a couple and with their children before becoming a blended family. I was pleased when they took my advice.

The counseling took more time and cost more than they expected because the counselor uncovered serious issues to which they had been blind. One day, when Debbie brought one of her children in to be treated for an ankle injury, she seemed irritated with me. As we talked she expressed her displeasure with my recommendation that they go to a counselor. I listened and then reassured her that this investment in time and treasure would pay a handsome dividend. It would, I emphasized, probably save time and money in the future. She shook her head in disbelief.

"Debbie," I asked, "Would you be willing to accept my recommendation in faith and see it through?"

She nodded.

They did see the process through. Barb and I attended their wedding. I continued to care for the family until I left my practice. We lost touch for several years, but then Scott sent me a letter. I share a part of it with you:

> I know so many other families that didn't follow our path. Most have now gone through a second divorce. But not us! The counseling gave us skills and tips we have used every day since. Walt, I'm not saying the path was easy, but without these skills it might have been impossible. Thanks for caring enough to insist we trek down this road less traveled!

If we parents are to raise highly healthy children, we must work on having highly healthy marriages and families in which to nurture them. We all need to work continually on improving the health of our relationships with God, our spouse, and our children. And we *all* can improve. Some of us have more difficult circumstances and greater challenges than others, but every one of us can and must take steps to make our families as healthy as possible—for the health of our children.

What about Adopted Children?

It may surprise you to hear that an adopted child may be at greater risk for not becoming highly healthy than a biological child in a two-parent family. In the United States, children living with adoptive parents are more than twice as likely to have a learning or behavioral problem as children living with their birth parents (36 percent versus 15 percent). A New Zealand study found that although adopted children in two-parent homes did significantly better than adopted children in single-parent homes, they were more likely to have higher rates of "externalizing behavior problems," such as behavior disorders, juvenile offending, and substance abuse.

Does this mean parents shouldn't adopt children? Absolutely not! Every child is precious in God's eyes and deserves the chance to be loved. The Bible places a special emphasis on the value of orphaned children. God himself adopts us as his children. Adoption affords the opportunity for a couple to come alongside a child who needs physical, emotional, and spiritual nurturing. Adopting and caring for orphans is one of the most sacrificial, loving things a couple can do.

Do keep in mind, though, the unique issues that can greatly influence a child's health. Some boys and girls who were abused or unloved prior to adoption react to those painful experiences in a variety of negative ways. Others struggle with identity problems and wonder why their "real" mothers and fathers didn't want them. Once they become adolescents, many are driven to find their biological parents.

As with many other behavioral issues, the critical factors are each child's particular temperament and the ways in which he or she is loved, nurtured, and raised by his or her parents. A 1985 study of forty-four families with biological children only, forty-five with adopted children only, and forty-four with biological and adopted children showed that adoptive placement of a child in a mixed family does not affect the biological child's overall adjustment and may, in fact, have positive effects on the adopted child. In general, a child does much better in a two-parent adoptive home than in a single-parent home. Adoptive children living with unmarried mothers are more likely to have a wide range of poor health measures. My deepest hope is that highly healthy parents won't be reluctant to adopt children because they're afraid of the problems that might develop. As I've tried to make clear, *every* child has unique challenges; *every* child is difficult to raise. Without a doubt, *every* child requires all the creative energy and skill a parent can muster. But *every* child is worth the effort, and there is no higher calling than to do an excellent job of raising highly healthy children.

THE MEANEST MOM IN THE WORLD

I'll conclude this chapter with a story about our family. Barb and I worked hard to have a highly healthy marriage—and we took very seriously our job of learning to be good parents and to raise highly healthy children. But there were times when we failed and didn't do the best we could have. There were times when we were doing the best we could, but we wondered if we were succeeding.

When Scott was in middle school, we were having dinner one evening when he commented, "Mom, I think you're the meanest mom in the world."

He kept eating, but Barb, Kate, and I paused in mid-bite. His voice and tone hadn't been mean-spirited—it was more matter-of-fact than anything.

"What did you say?" inquired an incredulous Kate.

He looked up and smiled. Then he reached into his pocket and pulled out an article and read it to us. Here's what he read:

The Meanest Mother

I had the meanest mother in the whole wide world. While other kids ate candy for breakfast, we had to have cereal, eggs, or toast. When others had cokes and candy for lunch, I had to eat a sandwich. And you can guess, my supper was different than the other kids' also. But at least I wasn't alone in my sufferings. My sister and two brothers had the same mean mother as I did.

My mother insisted on knowing where we were at all times. You'd think we were on a chain gang. She had to know who our friends were and where we were going. She insisted if we said we'd be gone an hour, that we be gone one hour or less—not one hour and one minute. I am ashamed to admit it, but she actually struck us. Not once, but each time we had a mind of our own and did as we pleased. That poor belt was used more on our seats than it was to hold up Daddy's pants. Can you imagine someone actually hitting a child just because he disobeyed. Now you can begin to see how mean she really was.

We had to wear clean clothes and take a bath. The other kids always wore their clothes for days. We reached the height of insults because she made our clothes herself, just to save money. Why, oh why, did we have to have a mother who made us feel different from our friends? The worst is yet to come.

We had to be in bed by nine each night and up at eight the next morning. We couldn't sleep till noon like our friends. So while they slept, my mother actually had the nerve to break the child-labor law. We had to wash dishes, make beds, learn to cook and all sorts of cruel things. I believe she laid awake at night thinking of mean things to do to us.

She always insisted upon us telling the truth, the whole truth, and nothing but the truth, even if it killed us—and it nearly did. By the time we were teenagers, she was much wiser, and our life became even more unbearable. None of this tooting the horn of a car for us to come running. She embarrassed us to no end by making our dates and friends come to the door to get us. If I spent the night with a girlfriend, can you imagine she checked on me to see if I was really there. I never had the chance to elope to Mexico. That is if I'd had a boyfriend to elope with. I forgot to mention, while my friends were dating at the mature age of 12 and 13, my old-fashioned mother refused to let me date until the age of 15 and 16. Fifteen, that is, if you dated only to go to a school function. And that was maybe twice a year.

Through the years, things didn't improve a bit. We could not lie in bed "sick" like our friends did, and miss school. If our friends had a toe ache, a hangnail, or serious ailment, they could stay home from school. Our marks in school had to be up to par. Our friends' report cards had beautiful colors on them, black for passing, red for failing. My mother, being as different as she was, would settle for nothing less than ugly black marks

As the years rolled by, first one and the other of us was put to shame. We were graduated from high school. With our mother behind us, talking, hitting, and demanding respect, none of us was allowed the pleasure of being a dropout.

My mother was a complete failure as a mother. Out of four children, a couple of us attained some higher education. None of us have ever been arrested, divorced, or beaten his mate. Each of my brothers served his time in the service of this country. And whom do we have to blame for the terrible way we turned out? You're right, our mean mother. Look at the things we missed. We never got to march in a protest parade, or to take part in a riot, burn draft cards, and a million and one other things that our friends did.

She forced us to grow up into God-fearing, educated, honest adults. Using this as a background, I am trying to raise my three children. I stand a little taller and I am filled with pride when my children call me mean.

Because, you see, I thank God He gave me the meanest mother in the whole world.

While Scott was reading, Barb reached under the table to hold my hand. Before he was done, tears were streaming down her cheeks. Tears were filling my eyes, too.

When he was done, Scott folded the paper and put it down. He looked at me and commented, "You're pretty mean yourself."

We all laughed.

That night, before we went to sleep, Barb and I had a moment of prayer. We were thankful for our children. We were thankful for the wisdom we had gained by trying to learn the skills and trying to make the sacrifices necessary to be the parents of highly healthy children. We were thankful to have grown up in nurturing family relationships. We were delighted to provide the same for Kate and Scott—and we're pleased they're now such neat young adults.

Chapter Eight

Establish a Spiritual Foundation

A five-year-old girl was sitting on her mother's lap, enjoying a time of quiet conversation. Her mother prayed with and for her child, read her Bible stories each evening, and took her to worship services frequently, so it wasn't surprising when the girl asked, "Mom, does God live in your heart?"

The mother smiled and nodded affirmatively.

Wanting to find out more, the girl asked, "Can I listen?" Her mother laughed as the daughter placed her head against her chest. Suddenly the little girl's eyes widened, and she jerked her head away.

"Did you hear anything?" the mother asked.

"I did!" the daughter exclaimed. "God was making coffee!"

Observant parents soon understand that a child, like an adult, is a spiritual being. Every child is created in God's likeness, God's image, and has the capacity for a personal relationship with him. A child can learn to see life through spiritual eyes and apply spiritual truths in ways that deeply affect his or her beliefs and choices. The earlier this spiritual foundation is laid, the more likely it is to thrive during adulthood.

A SPIRITUAL FOUNDATION IS ESSENTIAL

A strong spiritual foundation is an essential component of highly healthy children, families, and society. Children who have a healthy spiritual foundation grow up knowing they are created and loved by God, their Creator, who has endowed them with unique gifts, talents, and abilities. This foundation has an impact on every part of the child's life. It is a magnificent resource on which the child can draw for a lifetime.

When children have a personal connection with God—their Creator—and know what the Bible says about them, they are better equipped to accurately assess their abilities and gifts and live life to the fullest. In contrast, the failure to establish a healthy spiritual foundation can be a recipe for disaster. Although all children are born with a spiritual nature, a child who lacks a strong spiritual foundation and hasn't been shown how to have a personal relationship with God is at a huge disadvantage. Without a healthy, God-centered foundation and outlook, a child will likely struggle to figure out life and his or her place in it. Such a child may not realize how special each person is to the Creator and may fail to develop a healthy respect for all human life.

Consider for a moment Eric Harris and Dylan Klebold, the Columbine High School shooters. Their autopsies reportedly showed they were healthy physically. However, their emotional and social health wheels were severely damaged, and their spiritual wheel was totally deflated. According to videotapes the killers made weeks before America's most deadly high school shooting, they shared an intense hostility toward Christianity and Christians. They obviously had no respect for human life, as demonstrated by their brutal murder of twelve classmates and one teacher before taking their own lives.

Many people have asked why kids commit such senseless and violent acts. Explanations range from access to guns to mental disorders. Many variables, including some explored in this book, contribute to children being highly unhealthy. But there are three characteristics that repeatedly emerge in the research: spiritual emptiness, a toxic social environment, and family instability. Dr. James Garbarino, who has conducted many interviews with juvenile murderers, claims that when these three characteristics come together, they form a lethal mixture that is especially unhealthy and harmful to children. He calls this spiritual emptiness in children a "crisis of meaninglessness." I describe it as a "spiritual vacuum," or the lack of a healthy spiritual foundation.

Dr. Garbarino's research leads him to conclude that a lack of spiritual meaning in a child's life leads to despair and plays an important role in the lives of violent juveniles. He writes, "With neither hope nor a sense of purpose, troubled [children] are psychologically adrift and . . . are drawn to nihilism, Satanism, and all the other 'isms' of the dark side." Without a sense that their lives have a higher purpose grounded in a religious faith based on true spirituality (which I'll explain shortly), some of these children will see no point in restraining offensive or violent behavior.

Garbarino's findings concur with what I saw during my two decades of medical practice. Children who lacked a spiritual foundation often lived by the simple creed, "I am born; I live; I die." At best, the only values spiritually empty children receive from our culture are materialism and the pursuit of physical pleasure. Thus the best-understood purposes for existence are to accumulate "things" (such as power, possessions, and position) and to fulfill desires for the "Killer Bs" (beauty, brawn, and bucks). When these desires are not fulfilled (or when they are fulfilled but not accompanied by satisfaction or significance) *and* there is no spiritual foundation to mitigate the resulting emptiness, confusion, frustration, or hostility, the result can be worse than unhealthy; it can be deadly.

Research by psychologist Andrew Weaver links religious and spiritual experience to children's behavior and development. He concludes that a spiritual foundation helps to buffer children from the cultural and social poisons of modern life. He found many studies documenting the anchoring effect of a spiritual foundation. Religious belief among children has many healthy outcomes including reduced suicide attempts, less depression, better response to trauma, and less substance abuse. Other research shows that religious faith can give children a sense of hope and a higher purpose in life. There simply is no substitute for a healthy spiritual foundation in the life of a highly healthy child.

Pam and Jim Royal learned this the hard way. After they were married, they chose me to be their family physician. My initial examination included a spiritual assessment, from which I learned they had no church background and were fairly hostile toward spiritual matters. Jim told me, "I have no interest in such fairy tales. I'm interested in things that are real." Nevertheless, they knew of my faith and seemed to tolerate it. Pam once told me, "For a religious person, you're a pretty good guy!"

I kept the Royals on my prayer list for years. I delivered their three beautiful children but could not sway them from many of their unhealthy decisions. Pam and Jim fully devoted themselves to their careers. They lived in one of the nicest homes in town, drove new cars and SUVs, wore the best clothes, and took international vacations and expensive cruises—and they left their children in day care many hours each weekday and with family or friends on weekends.

The children lacked nothing materially. When I saw them for well-child visits, they wore the nicest clothes and had the best handheld electronics. However, in my opinion they were deprived of a healthy emotional, relational, and spiritual foundation. And, as you're beginning to see, homes built without these healthy foundations crumble easily.

Problems surfaced during the children's preteen and teen years. The oldest boy, who began abusing alcohol while young, got into fights and threw tantrums at school. The middle girl wrestled with a terrible self-image and immersed herself in drugs and sexual experimentation. The youngest daughter became enamored with Goth culture and attempted suicide at age twelve.

How did their parents respond? They just bought the children more things. They sent them to expensive summer camps where they interacted with and learned from children of other dysfunctional families. They put the children into therapy and pushed to get them on medications. They meted out harsh punishment, which produced anger and backlash. They blamed the school, its teachers, and me for failing them.

But one day Jim Royal entered my office, distraught and almost inconsolable. "Dr. Walt," he said, wiping away tears, "I've really messed up my life and my family. I want to change."

"What's going on?" I asked.

Jim explained that for some time his life and marriage had been on the rocks. His family was highly dysfunctional. His children were violent, addicted, and depressed. He had professional success but no satisfaction. Even worse, he felt his life had no significance. All these factors led him to accept a friend's invitation to attend a luncheon where a highly successful businessman explained why men need to build a spiritual foundation. During the talk, Jim learned how a personal relationship with God had changed this man's career, marriage, and relationship with his children.

"I couldn't help but think of you," Jim explained. "For years and years you've encouraged Pam and me to lay down a spiritual foundation for our marriage and our children. Sometimes you'd make me angry when you would suggest it. But I've watched you in your practice and with your family in the community. You have something we don't have." He paused, then continued, "It's time for me to begin to build that foundation. I just hope it's not too late."

That very day Jim began to make changes. Barb and I met with him and Pam weekly to discuss some of the things we had learned during our spiritual journey, and we were delighted when the couple began attending church with us. Jim's and Pam's change of heart and their efforts to build a spiritual foundation resulted in many changes in their lives and their children's lives.

Let me be clear, this process wasn't easy. It took lots of work. There were setbacks and difficulties. But slowly and surely, Jim, Pam, and their children began changing in remarkable ways. When I left my practice to join Focus on the Family, the whole family attended my going-away party. It was an emotional parting. I felt so blessed to have been used by God in the remarkable transformation of this precious family. Once bordering on destruction and tinkering with evil, they chose a new direction and were changed indeed.

When Jim found out I was writing this book, he called me and said, "Walt, let dads know that I just wish I had come to my senses earlier! Building a foundation is easiest if you start early. We were almost too late. If our children had not been able to watch their dad and mom begin to grow spiritually, if they had not heard us apologize to them for our many mistakes, if they had not been able to see our "love if" become "love in spite of"—well, I'm not sure what would have happened. Our children were on the edge of living lives with the potential for much harm, maybe even evil. Our family and our family's future really were rescued."

WHAT KIND OF SPIRITUAL FOUNDATION DO CHILDREN NEED?

Without some sort of spiritual anchor, children end up adrift in a toxic society that provides no real answers to their searching questions about the meaning of life. Tragically, our culture has become increasingly hostile to religion and religious beliefs. Rather than emphasizing the importance of true spirituality and life-changing religious faith, most cultural institutions today no longer encourage and support spiritual health. Academicians have denounced true spirituality. Hollywood has mocked it. Legislative activism and judicial tyranny have virtually banned it from the public square.

As a result, spiritual, religious, and moral themes have been summarily drummed out of most public school curriculums. Some students have been banned from reading their Bibles in school, and student-initiated religious groups have been blocked from meeting on school grounds. Some public schools are even wary of affirming such universal values as respect, responsibility, caring, and honesty for fear that they may be accused of promoting the values of a particular religion.

Ironically, true spirituality—the very prescription that shows the most promise in preventing unhealthiness and treating highly unhealthy children— is considered by many people to be irrelevant and even harmful. As a result, many children have no spiritual foundation at home. They lack a spiritual anchor. They're in a crisis of meaninglessness, and they have few remedies that will get them out of it.

But there is good news. Children hunger to fill their spiritual vacuum. After the Columbine and 9/11 tragedies, students sought comfort as they flocked to religious leaders and religious institutions. These children wanted more than grief counseling; they wanted spiritual hope and meaning. Many of them found what they needed in the context of a larger, transcendent story that only true spirituality can provide.

So what is true spirituality? Among the definitions for spirituality and other related words (such as faith, morality, and religion), the concept of *true spirituality*, or what some researchers call *intrinsic spirituality*, is clearly outlined in the Bible. True spirituality is distinguished from faith, morality, or religion in that it involves an authentic, growing, personal relationship with a personal God. This relationship is not bound by race, ethnicity, economic status, or class. It always promotes the wellness and welfare of others and of self. It includes the beliefs and values by which an individual lives, and it results in the visible spiritual fruit of love, joy, peace, patience, kindness, goodness, faithfulness, gentleness, and self-control.

I'm not alone in recognizing the benefits of true spirituality in highly healthy children. According to many other researchers, children and adults

My Discovery of True Spirituality

My brothers and I grew up with parents who took us to church nearly every Sunday. I served as an altar boy and attended church camps. Although I learned much about religion, I had no personal relationship with God. I first realized this in college when I began to wrestle with the meaning of life and my own nagging sense of meaninglessness.

Some guys in my fraternity house claimed to have found meaning, joy, and satisfaction through a personal relationship with God through Jesus Christ. I had never heard of such a thing! One day, I asked my friend Rich to tell me more about this relationship with God. He explained that all humans make mistakes; they do wrong things they wished they could take back, or they make mistakes they wish they had never made. I could identify with that! The problem was, the wrongs, mistakes, and dishonest actions in my past placed me in a position where I was separated from God and could not have a personal relationship with him. When Rich told me this, I knew in my heart it was true.

But then, almost as though he read my mind, Rich told me that God also deeply loved me, and because of that love God had sent Jesus Christ—his Son—to live a perfect life with no wrongdoing and to die on the cross for all *my* wrongdoing. Rich explained that Jesus' death paid the penalty that God demanded for all my wrongs—past and future. He told me I could not earn this and would never deserve it; it was simply a free gift from God.

If I accepted that gift, Rich explained, then God would forgive all my wrongdoing. My life could start over again, with a personal relationship with God that would result in love, joy, peace, patience, kindness, goodness, faithfulness, gentleness, and self-control. I tell you, those were some of the things I desperately needed in my life.

Finally, Rich explained that I could begin that relationship any time I wanted to. All I had to do was have a private talk with God. Rich said I just needed to admit to God that I had done wrong things and that I knew I didn't have a personal relationship with him. Then Rich told me to ask God to forgive me so I could begin a new relationship with him.

That night, I turned off the light in my room and said a prayer very similar to this: "Dear God. I know I haven't been living my life for you. I know I've done much wrong in my life. I'm asking you to forgive me of all the wrong I've done. I believe you sent your Son, Jesus, to die for me on the cross to pay the penalty for my wrongdoing. I want to turn from my corrupt nature and follow you. I invite you to come into my heart and life. In Jesus' name. Amen."

There were no fireworks, and I didn't hear any angels singing. I just went to sleep. But I kept my commitment to God to read his word (the Bible) and talk to him daily.

My life has never been the same. My problems haven't magically disappeared. Like you, I have to deal with the daily struggles and hassles of life. But this personal relationship with God has given me joy, peace, and a deep satisfaction with life. I'm a different person and a different kind of physician. I've been a better husband and a much better parent. My faith has given me strength, but best of all, I know for a fact that when I face death, I'll spend eternity in heaven with my Creator.

who have a foundation of true spirituality frequently pray, apply the Bible's truths to daily life, believe they have a personal relationship with God, and practice what they preach. They are likely to testify to having a high level of satisfaction in life, a deep sense of well-being, and overall happiness. This kind of spirituality is associated with many positive physical, relational, and emotional health outcomes.

Not all spiritual foundations are equal, however. Research shows that different types of spiritual foundations have different effects. Consider the following:

- Certain types of faith and spirituality, religious beliefs, and activities may even harm our health. I call this *negative spirituality* (or religiousness). Religion that separates people from community and family, encourages blind devotion and obedience to a single charismatic leader, or promotes religious healing to the exclusion of research-based medical care, for example, is likely to adversely affect health. It may even prevent children (and adults) from becoming highly healthy.

- The way in which we practice our spirituality affects our health. Research reveals that the benefits of spirituality are less significant when people merely go through the motions of religious tradition or use religion in self-serving, utilitarian ways. Researchers call this *extrinsic spirituality*. People who only attend worship services and programs in their religious community tend to experience an external faith that is less likely to be associated with positive health outcomes.

- Religion that fosters true, positive, intrinsic spirituality is likely to be highly healthy, in contrast to religion that is negative or fosters extrinsic spirituality only. This helps to explain why true spirituality is such a powerful force in regulating behavior. An individual who pursues true spirituality lives out a moral value system that typically results in positive or healthy outward behavior.

Look back at the Columbine High School shootings, and you'll see a dramatic example of the difference between true spirituality and extrinsic spirituality. According to her friends and parents, student Cassie Bernall was well on her way to the "dark side." She reportedly was troubled and withdrawn, dabbling in witchcraft, and becoming increasingly isolated. Lacking true spirituality, she was attempting to fill her spiritual vacuum with a false and dark spirituality. Her downward path, however, was halted by a spiritual conversion two years prior to the shootings. Her newfound faith, stemming from true spirituality, resulted in dramatic life changes that removed her from a potentially destructive course.

Evidently Cassie's dramatic change from spiritual darkness to spiritual light, which included praying and reading her Bible, had angered Eric Harris and Dylan Klebold. As they approached her, one of them asked, "Do you believe in God?"

Without hesitation, Cassie replied, "Yes."

"Why?" she was asked.

But before she could answer, she was shot in the head.

Her story shows the power of a spiritual foundation to help anchor a child's life and turn it from being highly unhealthy to becoming highly healthy. Her killers, on the other hand, had deeply immersed themselves in a different kind of spirituality. They embraced the dark elements of Nazism and the nihilism of Nietzsche, and they consumed a steady diet of death-themed music, films, and video games.

The spiritual foundation we help our children establish is the primary motivator that enables them to resist evil and choose healthy behavior. Because every person is created to have a healthy relationship with God, it is impossible for a child to become highly healthy without a solid spiritual foundation. It's up to us as parents to help lay this foundation. The stakes for not doing so are high.

A foundation of true spirituality is associated with many healthy outcomes physically, emotionally, and relationally. I'm fascinated by the large number of scientific studies showing that people who have a spiritual foundation cope better with physical and mental illness. People with greater religious involvement have been shown to have less depression and to recover more quickly than people with less religious involvement. Although a spiritual foundation doesn't guarantee physical health, the impact of a strong spiritual faith, devout prayer, and religious socialization has far-reaching consequences that are, I believe, greatly underestimated. Spiritual beliefs and prayer apparently help patients— adults and children alike—cope better with illness and result in less stress, anxiety, and depression and in greater social support. These effects counteract the many stress-related physiological changes that can impair healing. Research has shown that religious involvement is related to stronger immune functioning, lower blood pressure, lower levels of stress hormones, and longer survival. In the case of catastrophic trauma or illness, a person with a foundation of true spirituality generally recovers better and is better able to cope with medical conditions that aren't improving.

Do you remember little Daryl, the boy with end-stage cancer I wrote about in chapter 1? One day as we chatted, I asked, "Daryl, what makes you the most happy?"

I was thinking he'd mention the ice cream parlor at Give Kids the World, his visit with Disney characters, or his morning at Disney World or Sea World.

He thoughtfully replied, "It's being able to talk to God in prayer."

I smiled and asked, "Does he talk back?"

Daryl looked at me as though I had two heads. "Of course! He talks to me in my thoughts. He walks with me into surgeries and procedures. He holds me when I cry. He's always with me."

I was stunned by the faith of this wise little boy.

Daryl then looked up at me and asked, "Dr. Walt, know what makes me sad?"

"What, Daryl?" I asked, trying to blink away tears.

"It's the little boys and girls here who don't know God—who don't know that heaven is going to be so much cooler than here."

Daryl's spiritual foundation provided him with incredible resources in dealing with his cancer. In fact, his highly healthy emotional, relational, and spiritual wheels made him more highly healthy than most of the patients I met during more than twenty years of medical practice.

NURTURING OUR CHILDREN'S SPIRITUAL HEALTH

As a parent, I want to fulfill my God-given role of nurturing my children so that they enjoy the high level of spiritual health Daryl demonstrated to me. I know from my years of medical practice that nearly every parent wants the same. I delivered more than 1,500 babies, yet I can count on one hand the pregnant moms I cared for who did not think about spiritual things during pregnancy. When a mom feels her baby move in the womb, when a dad first feels the kick of his baby through his wife's abdominal wall, when parents and siblings catch their first glimpse of a baby on an ultrasound, they are almost always awestruck. It's a profound moment when we realize the miracle of life growing in the womb—sometimes terrifying, sometimes exciting, but always awesome and mysterious. We almost always sense that something divine is happening. I often heard parents exclaim, "O my God!" while looking at their babies on ultrasound. They expressed their subconscious recognition that something very special had happened—the creation of new life—and it turned their thoughts toward spiritual things.

The Bible explains why we respond this way: "But the basic reality of God is plain enough. Open your eyes and there it is! By taking a long and thoughtful look at what God has created, people have always been able to see what their eyes as such can't see: eternal power, for instance, and the mystery of his divine being."

Truly the birth of a child makes us aware of God. To ensure that my patients—parents and parents-to-be—understood the importance of building a healthy spiritual foundation for their children, I talked with them about it. I encouraged them to assess their spiritual health and decide how they were going to pass on a healthy, true, intrinsic spirituality to their children. I'm still sharing the same message today—through my books, on radio and television, and in my public speaking.

Yet I'm deeply grieved when I hear of the many parents who do little or nothing to nurture a spiritual foundation for their children. A 2002 national survey asked parents in America if they believed religious faith to be important. A surprising 93 percent of parents felt religious faith was either "important" or "absolutely essential"; only 53 percent, however, felt they were succeeding in building a spiritual foundation for their children.

Sadly, many parents believe their children will "find" the spirituality they need on their own. Nothing could be further from the truth. Research shows that it becomes progressively more difficult to influence children spiritually as they grow older. A spiritual foundation established in childhood is much more likely to persist in adulthood. For example, researcher George Barna has shown that a young person who is not introduced to a personal relationship with God before the age of fourteen has little likelihood of developing such a relationship. According to Barna's survey, children ages five through thirteen have a 32 percent likelihood of beginning a personal relationship with God; children ages fourteen to eighteen have a 4 percent likelihood; adults from age nineteen until death have a 6 percent likelihood.

There is no doubt in my mind that a spiritual foundation is best taught and nurtured at an early age. Even very young children understand spiritual truth better than we realize. It is our privilege and responsibility as parents to build a strong spiritual foundation for our children.

Dose of Wisdom

The top myth of parenting is that children should be free to choose their own belief system. This is like setting a boat out to sea without a rudder.

William Sears, M.D., pediatrician

SPIRITUAL TRAINING: IT'S A PARENT'S JOB

It's tempting to let others—youth pastors, pastors, priests, Sunday school teachers—give our children their spiritual training. Many parents believe that if they take their children to a church or synagogue to receive spiritual training from a pastoral professional or committed layperson, the children will "turn out all right." It may happen, but it's not nearly as life-changing or effective as when parents take charge of this God-given responsibility. Pastoral professionals may have more knowledge of spiritual things than a typical mom or dad, but they don't have—and aren't supposed to have—the heart-attachment parents have for their children. The average pastoral professional will never have the quality and quantity of time we parents should have with our children. A faith community can supplement the spiritual foundation laid at home, but it cannot replace it!

Furthermore, as parents, we are responsible for how our children are nurtured spiritually. We will not stand before the Lord and say, "It was my pastor's [or teacher's or ...] fault that my children didn't have a spiritual foundation." Children are God's gifts to us, and it is our job to parent our children—including setting their spiritual foundation. Granted, God has given us a serious responsibility. Phillip Johnson, executive director of Grace to You, captures the feelings of many parents when he makes this observation in an online essay: "Most Christian parents will admit to being somewhat intimidated by the weighty responsibility Scripture places on us. Our task is outlined in simple terms by verses like ... Ephesians 6:4: 'Bring [your children] up in the discipline and instruction of the Lord.' Understanding our solemn duty as parents *ought* to provoke a certain amount of fear and trembling." Despite the seriousness of our responsibility, Johnson goes on to offer great encouragement: "Then again, it needn't paralyze us. Teaching spiritual truth to children is a joy. No one is more receptive, more hungry to learn, or more trusting than a child. Chances are, you'll never find more eager disciples than your own children."

The Bible instructs us to teach our children spiritual truth, never hinting that children can't grasp God's Word. Johnson describes children as "better equipped now to assimilate spiritual truth than they will be when they are older. That's why Jesus called for childlike faith: 'Truly I say to you, whoever does not receive the kingdom of God like a child shall not enter it at all.'"

I can't overemphasize how important it is for parents not only to teach but to model spiritual faith and to be willing to be taught by their children. Parents who practice their faith from the heart are much more likely to have children who do the same. Jim and Pam Royal, whom I spoke of earlier, illustrate this. Pam had sensed that their children needed some sort of spiritual foundation, so although the couple's weekend travels and activities kept them from attending church, Pam sometimes arranged for her children's caregivers to take them to church. When the children were young, they attended vacation Bible school at a local church. When Pam realized that such religious activities weren't altering her children's downward spiral, however, she gave up on church and spiritual things.

Everything changed when Pam committed herself to a personal relationship with God. When *she* began praying for her husband and children, when *she* began reading the Bible daily, when *she* began going to church, when *her* life began to change spiritually from the inside out, her children were influenced more deeply than she ever could have hoped for. As she and Jim changed for the better, their children wanted those spiritual changes in their lives as well.

The Royals' experience in modeling true spirituality for their children is a lesson the Bible has proclaimed for centuries. Moses clearly understood the importance of modeling spiritual teaching. Notice his clear emphasis that the responsibility for building our children's spiritual foundation rests on us, their parents:

> *Hear, O Israel: The LORD our God, the LORD is one. Love the LORD your God with all your heart and with all your soul and with all your strength. These commandments that I give you today are to be upon your hearts. Impress them on your children. Talk about them when you sit at home and when you walk along the road, when you lie down and when you get up. Tie them as symbols on your hands and bind them on your foreheads. Write them on the doorframes of your houses and on your gates.*

These verses were a true guide for Barb and me. From them we learned that *we*—not someone else—were the people God intended to teach spiritual truth to our children. Their primary religious training facility was to be *our home,* not a church. As important as it is to pray with our children each night, it's even more important to live and teach our children spiritual truth all day long. References to God and expressions of our spiritual beliefs should permeate our conversation and interactions with our children. It should be obvious that our love for God is the first priority in our lives.

Dr. James Dobson minces no words in emphasizing the importance of teaching spiritual truth to our children: "The reason this is such a critical responsibility is that the world will be giving your children very different messages in the days ahead. It will take them to hell if not counterbalanced by a firm spiritual foundation at home. This is one task about which we can't afford to be lackadaisical."

Our efforts to teach and live out our faith in our children's presence have far more impact than we can imagine. Barb and I caught a glimpse of this when our family spent a Thanksgiving Day in Washington, D.C., where Kate was a White House intern. We ate Thanksgiving dinner in the gigantic, ornate lobby of Union Station. As we've done in the past, we shared things for which we were grateful. For some reason Kate and Scott, now in college, began mentioning meaningful childhood memories. With tears in our eyes, Barb and I held hands and listened as they blessed us in ways they couldn't even imagine.

Later that evening, Barb and I reflected on the incredible gift our children spontaneously presented to us.

"Did you notice," Barb inquired, "how many of their memories involved church or our family's spiritual activities?"

Suddenly it hit me. "Yes!" I exclaimed. Establishing a healthy spiritual wheel during childhood is likely to result in highly healthy children. And a child's spiritual foundation starts, first and foremost, with the spiritual health of his or her parents. That night, Barb and I discussed some of the things we intentionally did to provide Kate and Scott with a spiritual foundation.

ESTABLISHING YOUR CHILD'S SPIRITUAL FOUNDATION

We believe you can take some important steps to establish your child's spiritual foundation. Let me share several with you as I bring this chapter to a conclusion.

Balance Your Own Spiritual Wheel

I'm convinced God wants us, as parents, to be as physically, emotionally, relationally, and spiritually healthy as possible. He wants us to enjoy healthy relationships with others. Most of all, he wants us to have a healthy relationship with him. The best way I know to become a highly healthy person is to develop a true spirituality that results in the most important and enduring form of health and vitality.

So how does your spiritual wheel look? Is it fully inflated, and is it bouncing along in proper balance and alignment? Or is it a little flat? Maybe you haven't maintained it for a long time, and it's taken a beating from the nails you've picked up along the road of life. Or maybe, on careful examination, you've realized you're riding on the spare and have tossed the spiritual wheel in the trunk!

Medical studies clearly show that spiritual distress can negatively affect physical, emotional, and relational health. Spiritual distress or crisis occurs when people cannot find meaning, hope, joy, satisfaction, love, peace, comfort, strength, and connection in life. It also occurs when tension exists between what their beliefs are and what's happening in their lives. So if you're a bit flat or off track, or even if you just need a maintenance check, I recommend the self-test developed by George Barna.

The questions on this list are designed to help you determine how well you are doing in your personal spiritual journey. Based on Barna's two decades of research on spiritual development and fulfillment, the questions focus on key factors involved in spiritual health. Although no evaluation tool can perfectly assess every dimension of your spiritual life, your responses can provide insight into your spiritual condition. As you work through this assessment, be honest. Its value lies in helping you identify strengths and weaknesses, which can then lead you to a more focused and meaningful spiritual journey.

BARNA SPIRITUAL JOURNEY ASSESSMENT

Developed and provided by George Barna, Barna Research Group, Ltd., Ventura, California

How true is this characteristic of you?

1 = Not at all or never

4 = Often or usually

2 = Not much or rarely

5 = Completely or always

3 = Somewhat or occasionally

1. You maintain an intense level of respect, awe, humility, and gratitude toward God—in acknowledgment of his superiority and perfection. _____

2. You effectively share the substance of your faith with people who have an interest in it. _____

3. You pray for the needs and future of others. _____

4. The choices and decisions you make are based on spiritual principles and values. _____

5. Your speech and behavior pleases God. _____

6. When you pray, you both speak and listen to God. _____

7. Worship is not just an event you attend—you try to live your life as an act of worship to God. _____

8. You are held morally and spiritually accountable by others who know and care for you. _____

9. You give away your time, abilities, and money sacrificially for the benefit of the needy. _____

10. You fight injustice and inequality. _____

11. You strive to live out the "Golden Rule"—to love other people as you want them to love you. _____

12. Your attitudes, values, and thoughts please God. _____

Total _____

Add up your score. A score of forty-eight or higher indicates you are likely to be spiritually healthy; a score of twenty-four or lower indicates you may not be spiritually healthy.

Did your score on the questionnaire surprise you? If it was lower than you expected or want it to be, look for two or three things you can do, starting right now, to improve your spiritual health. Your children's health and the health of your future grandchildren depend on it. If you can't think of anything to do, make an appointment with a pastoral counselor who can help you in this area. Or pick up a copy of *Becoming a Highly Healthy Person*. In this book I've provided measures you can use to calibrate your physical, emotional, relational, and spiritual wheels. You can order a copy or learn more at www.highlyhealthy.net.

Teach Your Children Spiritual Truth Daily

It's up to you to serve your family a healthy portion of spiritual teaching every day. Some days you may serve a small—or large—portion, but children need God's Word every day. Your children are much less likely to grow and mature spiritually if you don't feed them. Are you relying on "spiritual experts" to feed your children? Are you waiting and hoping they'll pick up spiritual truth later in life? Or are you leading them in a daily time of family worship and Bible reading that will help you accomplish your goal?

Nurturing your children's spiritual foundation doesn't have to be—and shouldn't be—boring. Spiritual truth can be taught with songs and stories. Prayer time before family meals and at bedtime communicates spiritual belief and practice. Worship as a family. Schedule family Bible time, just as you schedule bath or nap times. There are many wonderful resources available for parents who wish to help their child begin to form a strong spiritual foundation.

Resource Box   **Helpful Hints**

Practical Tips for Spiritual Teaching

No child is too young to learn from the most important book in history. To help you communicate its message to your children, I've included several great suggestions from author and mother Lynne Thompson.

- *Set a routine for Bible time.* Try to have it at approximately the same time each day, perhaps after breakfast or before snack time.
- *Sing fun songs.* Bible songs on cassette or CD can get you started. Enjoy clapping and jumping.
- *Read from a children's Bible.* Use a toddler or picture Bible. Keep the stories short. Some children enjoy holding the Bible while you read. Using a puppet to tell the Bible story is always a treat.
- *Introduce additional material.* Bible coloring books are a great way to share a story. You may want to read holiday books that depict spiritual stories.

- *Toss in real life.* If the Bible story contains any objects you have in your home, use them. Visual aids make the story real to a child. If you're reading about Noah's ark, pull the cushions off the couch to make a boat, then bring aboard all the stuffed animals.
- *Include a memory verse.* For older children, pick a verse from the Bible and repeat it each day until your child memorizes it. Practice by allowing her to fill in a word you leave out. Reward with a sticker, then move on to another verse.
- *Make prayer easy.* In the beginning, you'll have to model a simple prayer. For example, "Thank you, God, for sunshine. Thank you for today. Amen." After a while, ask your child if there's something he'd like to pray for.
- *Be patient.* Bible time may occasionally have to be cut short due to a sleepy child or a bad day. The goal is to stay committed to providing as much of a positive Bible routine as possible. It will become a part of your child's day that says, "Let's take time to have fun with God!"

Pray with and for Your Children and Family

In *The Successful Child*, pediatrician and parenting expert William Sears writes, "Many parents devote a great deal of effort to shaping their child's intellectual, emotional, or physical development, but they shy away from teaching spirituality. They are neglecting a critical tool for success. Prayer also makes belief more real and shapes the identity of a family." Family prayer, he says, teaches your children what you believe. Prayer also "teaches empathy," he notes, "especially as siblings pray for each other."

I couldn't agree more. Loving parents who are spiritually healthy would not even try to raise children without praying for them regularly and praying with them often. As you can tell from the stories I tell about myself, I'm not always the best dad or spouse. More times than I care to admit, I've made big mistakes as a parent. Yet I believe that Barb's and my prayers for ourselves, each other, and our children are one of the most important tools we have as parents.

Barb and I know Kate and Scott better than anyone in the world, so we are the very best candidates to pray for their needs. Our consistent prayers for them were an incredible encouragement and comfort to them. Dr. James Dobson expresses the importance of parenting with prayer more eloquently than I can. He writes, "Everything we do during those foundational child-rearing years should be bathed in prayer. There is not enough knowledge . . . to secure the outcome of our parenting responsibility without divine help. It is arrogant to think that we can shepherd our kids safely through the minefields of an increasingly sinful society. . . . Prayer is the key to everything."

Involve Your Family in a Faith Community

Parents best teach their children true spirituality when they practice as well as teach spiritual principles and do so in conjunction with the presence and care of a larger faith community. Involvement in a faith community can provide many documented spiritual health benefits:

- Children who attend church when they are young tend to continue regular church attendance as adults (61 percent).
- About two out of three adults (63 percent) who were churched as children take their children to church, but only one in three adults (33 percent) who were unchurched as children take their children to church.
- Adults who attended church as children are twice as likely to read the Bible during a typical week as those who avoided churches when young and nearly 50 percent more likely to pray to God during a typical week.
- Adults who regularly attend worship services at churches or participate in other religious activities are more likely to be giving and volunteering members of their communities. Harvard University researcher Robert Putnam writes, "Faith communities in which people worship together are arguably the single most important repository of social capital in America."
- Regular participation in a faith community is highly healthy socially. Putnam observes that regular worshipers and people who say that religion is very important to them are much more likely than other people to visit friends, to entertain at home, to attend club meetings, and to belong to a myriad of groups and organizations. What's more, says Putnam, people who join and attend churches regularly talk with 40 percent more people during the day than those who do not.

Prepare Your Children to Make a Difference in Their World

When I think of the potential of children who are highly healthy spiritually, I think first of Daryl, the little boy I met at Give Kids the World. His physical wheel was getting flatter because of the cancer ravaging his body, but his spiritual wheel was fully inflated and balanced. I greatly appreciate the lessons he unwittingly taught a young family physician about being highly healthy. He was a living example to me of what the Bible says: "For physical training is of some value, but godliness has value for all things, holding promise for both the present life and the life to come."

Daryl's "godliness," or spiritual foundation, gave him a great outlook for both this life and the life to come. Although his physical life would be short, his personal relationship with God was a tremendous resource to him and his family. When we parents build a healthy spiritual foundation for our children, it not only benefits them; it benefits the community and culture as well. The next chapters will focus on involving your children in suitable activities in the community and on cultivating their growth and maturity. A healthy spiritual foundation is critical for them as they go out into the world.

Chapter Nine

Connect with the Larger Community

Barb and I have always enjoyed visiting famous zoos. One day we visited a well-known animal park and watched one of the trained-animal shows. One of the more impressive acts was a huge eagle that had been trained to fly untethered around the open arena. A trainer described how this eagle had been blown out of its nest by a gunshot while it was still an eaglet. When hikers found the eaglet, it was blind in one eye and had a broken leg and wing. They brought it to the zoo for care.

The eaglet healed, but she was crippled and unable to survive in the wild. Her trainers wanted her to be as healthy as possible, so she needed to learn to fly. A cage was too small for her to fly around inside it, yet if she were released into the open and flew away, she could die.

So when the eaglet was young, the trainers began the process of letting her out with a tether on her leg. She would stretch and flap her wings. She learned to hop, walk, and fly while tethered to her trainers. As she grew, the trainers kept lengthening her tether as they taught her to respond to hand signals. They taught her how to make decisions about how and where to fly. Then, when she was ready, they let her fly into the open air without a tether.

Of course, this was a risk. The eagle could have flown away. Had she done so, she probably wouldn't have lived long. But having been "raised well" and having learned to trust her caregivers, she chose to return to them. Because the trainers had been willing to let her learn to fly—and then gave her the freedom to actually do it—she lived a much longer, healthier life than a caged eagle.

After the show, Barb and I talked about how the eagle symbolized the way we wanted to parent Kate and Scott. We wanted to teach them to fly, to interact successfully with the world around them. One day we would need to let them go—not too soon, but at the right time. Once we set them free, they would decide how and where to fly. Our job was to prepare them for flight.

GROWING BEYOND FAMILY

As important as family is in a child's development, children don't stay home forever—and they aren't supposed to. Children are meant to grow up and go out into the world, prepared to be highly healthy young adults—physically, emotionally, relationally, and spiritually. So it's our job as parents to nurture our children in such a way that they each discover their individual destinies and learn how to interact successfully in the world around them. Let's explore how we go about the process of guiding our children in their interactions with others so they can learn to fly freely.

A child's transition from family to the outside world begins at an early age. When our children are young, it's our job to choose the children and adults with whom they will interact. We also need to carefully choose those who will care for them in our absence. As our children mature, we lengthen the tether by guiding and advising as they choose friends and mentors. As their decisions become increasingly independent, we eventually reach a point where we release the tether and allow our children to make their own decisions about how and to whom they'll relate. Because these decisions affect our children's health in so many ways, it's important that we approach this aspect of parenting with great care.

During my years of medical practice, I noticed that parents tended to make one of two mistakes: They would keep the tether too short, or they'd release it too quickly. Children who are tethered too closely may pull against the tether in fits of rebellion. The tether, instead of keeping them close, causes them to pull away. Likewise, no tether—or too loose a tether—may prevent children from experiencing their parents' guidance and protection. Both mistakes are harmful to a child.

There are, of course, no firm and fast rules on how to lengthen or release the tether. Each child is unique, so our parenting should be different for each one. Those who trained the eagle had to be aware of these mistakes, too. Keeping the eagle tethered too long or releasing her too soon would have put her at risk and might have led to harm or even an early death.

Carl and Andee were college students during the late 1960s. Their parents were Depression-era children. Both their fathers were overly strict disciplinarians who would strike their children in anger. Both were tethered very, very tightly. As soon as they were able to escape, they did, and they vowed they'd parent differently from the way they were raised.

After a prolonged time of rebellion that included diving into the sexual revolution and drug experimentation, they chose to get married. They weren't sure why antisocial zealots such as themselves would turn to such an established social institution, but they did.

Before long they had three children. I was privileged to attend the birth of each child, an experience that was accompanied by flowers, aromatherapy, and New Age music. I was there for each child's well-child visits and sick care. But try as I would, I couldn't get Carl or Andee to use any discipline. Authority and rules were anathema to them.

"We won't do it!" Andee exclaimed to me one day. "It only harmed us, and we *won't* hurt our children."

Unfortunately, they failed to realize just how much they *were* injuring their children. Less than a decade later, after suffering through three horrendous teenage rebellions—including one teen wrestling with drug abuse and another who became an unwed mother, Andee came to see me in the midst of a severe depression. I explained her diagnosis and treatment options. She seemed dazed, turned to look out the window for a moment, then faced me with tears streaming down her cheeks.

"Dr. Walt," she confessed, " I just wish Carl and I had been better parents."

I gripped her hand, and my eyes also teared up. "Andee, how 'bout we start over, today."

She smiled and squeezed my hand. I couldn't help but think how much of her pain could have been avoided.

TEACHING OUR CHILDREN TO OBEY AND RESPECT AUTHORITY

Children who don't respect or know how to obey authority are destined for a rough ride in life. Unless your children learn how to submit to appropriate authority, they cannot be highly healthy because they won't be equipped to successfully interact in groups or in society as a whole. When we parents teach our children how to respond to appropriate authority when they are very young, we are preparing them for their future roles as husbands and wives, employees and employers, citizens and leaders.

Good habits such as obedience and respect for authority are not second nature to children; they require a lot of training. Children naturally resist and disobey authority. What child, for example, ever had to be taught how to say no? If we're honest, we adults naturally resist authority as well. Yet most children's habits, values (or morals), and beliefs tend to follow those they see their parents practice. When children see their parents fail to "practice what they preach" or "preach one thing and practice another," they tend to incorporate the behaviors they see into their lives.

I wish you could meet Abbie, Darla, and Corrie, the daughters of two of our closest friends. These young women are three of my favorite people. I met them when they were very young and have followed with much interest their growth and development through childhood, high school and college, and out into the world. To this day, when I talk to them in person or by phone, they always sprinkle "yes, sir" or "no, sir" throughout the conversation.

When they were young, their mom and dad taught them to respect and obey authority, a behavior the children saw in their parents' interactions with others. Their mom and dad understood that love must be balanced with limits. Love for a child fosters acceptance and appreciation. Limits foster accountability and respect for authority. Unconditional love and wise rules allow children to develop discipline and obedience, which are foundational to a child's emotional, relational, and spiritual health. Too much or too little of either or both can cause imbalance.

If there's anything that saddens me as I think of these three young ladies, it's that they are so unique. Although their behavior was the standard for children three decades ago, it is now uncommon, if not rare. Contemporary culture seems to bend over backward in allowing children to rebel against "good," God-given authority. By defying this authority, our children are told they can find their freedom, significance, satisfaction, and independence. But it just isn't the case. As my grandfather used to say, "Parents who fail to put their feet down usually have children who step on their toes!" Defying authority isn't healthy for individuals, and it isn't good for society.

Why are obedience to and respect for authority essential to a child's health and maturity? I believe it's because our Creator made us that way. Our Creator has given us an operation manual—the Bible—and it clearly teaches that it is highly healthy for boys and girls (as well as men and women) to be under authority: "Everyone must submit himself to the governing authorities, for there is no authority except that which God has established. The authorities that exist have been established by God. Consequently, he who rebels against the authority is rebelling against what God has instituted, and those who do so will bring judgment on themselves."

The "I want what I want when I want it" philosophy damages and can even destroy individuals and their relationships. In contrast to this philosophy, the Bible says, "Obey your leaders and submit to their authority . . . so that their work will be a joy, not a burden, for that would be of no advantage to you." Respecting and obeying God-given authority is healthy for the individual, and it brings joy to others.

Because Barb and I put great stock in the Bible's instructions, teaching Kate and Scott to respect and obey *God-ordained* authority was much more important to us than just teaching them to blindly obey *any* authority. The simplest way to teach this was to tell them that "bad," or "dangerous," authority would command what God forbids or forbid what God commands. We wanted them to know that it was right to say an emphatic no when someone told them to do what the Bible (or we) had taught them not to do. We wanted them to know that if someone told them *not* to do what was taught in the Bible, they should resist that authority. We wanted them to have an ethical, moral plumb line to carry in life—an ultimate authority—by which they could compare claims and commands.

So how can parents go about teaching respect for authority? Start young! Assign your children responsibilities that have real value. By assigning important work to Kate and Scott and teaching them how to do it, Barb and I demonstrated that their work was valuable and essential. (We avoided using the word *chores* because we felt it carried a negative connotation.) We started by giving them responsibility for such tasks as picking up their toys and putting dirty clothes in the hamper at ages two and three. By ages four and five, they had responsibility for putting away their washed clothes, hanging up towels after a bath, setting the table, and cleaning up after dinner. As they grew older, we kept teaching them to do more, and we trusted them to do it.

Child development experts tell us that children develop physical, intellectual, emotional, and relational skills as they gain confidence and competence in carrying out increasingly complex responsibilities. So as Kate and Scott completed tasks successfully, we bent over backward to thank and congratulate them. From time to time we offered a reward for a job that was especially well-done. We felt it was crucial to recognize their good work as a valuable contribution and to express this in front of one another, as well as in front of adult role models such as a neighbor, grandparent, youth pastor, or teacher. By working to catch Kate and Scott doing something well and by praising and encouraging them often, we could almost see their confidence grow.

We expected Kate and Scott to learn to overcome any obstacles that stood in the way of accomplishing tasks that had been assigned to them. We didn't allow excuses for not carrying out a job according to instructions. They could, of course, ask for further clarification if they didn't understand how to complete a particular job. We also expected them to act immediately, cheerfully, and diligently the first time a responsibility was assigned.

Teaching our children regular routines, including the assignment of household responsibilities, and following these routines ourselves is a great way we parents can establish consistent family guidelines for times of work and play. When we add generous helpings of encouragement, we not only nurture healthier children, we build healthier, happier households.

Resource Box   Helpful Hints

Training through Responsibility

Here are some ways parents can go about the process of assigning responsibilities to their children (adapted from the online article "Good Home Habits Taught Early On Have Long-Term Benefits"):

- Make a list, assign tasks, and stick to it. Assigning housework establishes a sense of teamwork and participation.
- Develop a weekly schedule for children and parents. It's crucial for each person to have an active role and sense of ownership in running the household.
- Allow children to be creative as they work, especially if they offer suggestions. There's usually more than one way to complete a specific task.
- Work side by side with your children whenever possible. It's a great opportunity to spend time together *and* get some work done! A good work ethic can be learned at an early age.
- Let your children imitate you. Encourage them to share in the same experiences and activities with which you

> may be engaged, even if it's as simple as using the phone
> or brushing your hair.
> - Spend more time in or around your home. When your
>   children learn to play and work in the home at an early
>   age, they value home as a haven later in life.
> - Reward a job well-done. Acknowledge and praise your
>   children's good work as a valuable contribution.

TEACHING OUR CHILDREN TO RESPECT THE DIFFERENCES THAT MAKE PEOPLE UNIQUE

As children venture out into the world, they will encounter people who look, speak, act, and believe differently from anyone they've ever known before. This can be highly unsettling. It can lead children to make critical or unfair judgments about others that may adversely affect their relationships throughout life. It's never too early, or too late, to encourage your children to accept and respect others.

Research shows that children between the ages of two and five become aware of differences in gender, culture, physical appearance, and functioning. Their curiosity leads them to ask questions such as, "Why is her skin so dark?" or, "Why does he speak funny?" They very quickly absorb the positive attitudes or negative biases attached to these differences by family members and other significant adults in their lives. Let me share an example.

While having dinner at a friend's home, one mom's five-year-old daughter leaned over and whispered, "Mommy, that lady isn't using good manners!"

Surprised, because "that lady" was a very proper and well-mannered British octogenarian, the mom asked, "What is it you noticed?"

In a disgusted tone, the little girl whispered, "Look how she uses her fork!"

"You're right!" the mom replied. "She doesn't hold her fork the way we do, but that's because she's lived most of her life in a different country, and their table manners aren't the same as ours. She is using exactly the table manners she was taught when she was little."

"Oh, I didn't know they could be different," the girl replied. In a short time, the girl and "that lady" became great admirers of one another.

If we want our children to like themselves and to cherish their uniqueness and to value diversity among people and cultures, we must learn how to help them resist biases based on gender, race, disability, culture, or social class.

These biases can create serious obstacles to healthy development. In order to be highly healthy, our children must learn how to interact fairly and productively with different types of people.

We parents must face and change our own biased attitudes in order to encourage our children's growth. It isn't enough to hide our own negative feelings or hope that our children won't notice. By our avoidance we may actually be teaching our children that some differences are not acceptable. In this area, as in many others, what we *do* makes all the difference.

When Kate and Scott were in elementary school, we had a dinner discussion about one of their Jewish friends. As we talked, Barb and I were surprised by some of the inaccurate perceptions our children harbored about our Jewish friends. They were also alarmingly uninformed about the Jewish roots of our own Christian heritage. So, we decided to celebrate the Jewish holidays for an entire year. During that year we came to understand, at least to a small degree, some crucial things about the Jewish faith. Our own faith was deepened in the process. Not only did our children's view of Judaism change, but their parents' view changed as well!

Resource Box   **Helpful Hints**

Teaching Respect for Our Differences

We live in a society where many biases exist, so we must actively counteract them. Here are some suggestions from the National Association for the Education of Young Children that will help you teach and model respect for others in daily life.

- Show no unfair bias in the friends, doctors, teachers, and other service providers you choose, or in the stores where you shop.
- Remember that what you do is as important as what you say.
- Teach your children that a person's appearance is never an acceptable reason for teasing or rejecting them. Immediately step in if you hear or see your child behave in such a way.
- Talk positively about each child's physical characteristics and cultural heritage. Help children learn the differences

between feelings of superiority and arrogance and feelings of self-esteem and pride in their own heritage.

- Provide opportunities for children to interact with other children who are racially or culturally different from themselves. Include in your family activities people who have various disabilities.

- Respectfully listen to and answer children's questions about differences they see. Don't ignore their questions, change the subject, or indicate that it's bad to ask such questions.

- Give your children tools to confront those who act against them because of bias or prejudice.

- Use accurate and fair images in contrast to stereotypes, and help your children think critically about what they see in books, movies, greeting cards, comics, and television ads and programs.

- Let children know that unjust things *can* be changed, and encourage them to take action.

TEACHING OUR CHILDREN TO CONTRIBUTE TO THE WORLD AROUND THEM

Have you ever received a suggestion that immediately made so much sense that you thought, "I wish I had thought of that"? That's what happened to me when Barb thought of a way to help ten-year-old Kate and seven-year-old Scott give of themselves to others—and gain a renewed sense of purpose in the process.

"Honey," she said to me, "I think I'd like the kids to come with us when you serve at the medical clinic for homeless people."

It was a brilliant idea!

Barb and I had helped establish a weekly medical clinic for homeless and uninsured people who lived in our town. It was an extension of our community soup kitchen and was supported by local churches. Doctors and nurses volunteered to examine patients, the local medical society donated money for low-cost prescription medications, and the hospitals provided needed services—all at no cost to our patients.

Barb and I were amazed when we brought Kate and Scott to the clinic. They pitched right in to help with the administrative work. They talked and laughed with the patients. Kate was a great listener. Scott was a tremendous conversationalist. Patients frequently commented on how much it meant to feel accepted and liked by our children.

Not only were Kate and Scott able to make a difference in the lives of other people; their volunteer service changed their view of themselves. They saw that they could make a difference in someone's life. They also saw how very blessed our family was in terms of health and worldly provisions.

Our family's experience isn't unique. According to experts, encouraging children to help out in their communities in meaningful ways is one of the healthiest activities parents can encourage them to do. To their credit, children tend to feel compassion for people in need and believe that if they help others, others will help them. Furthermore, children want to do something for a cause in which they believe.

Families—including children—have the power to make a huge difference in the lives of others and to make the world a better place. When families volunteer together, children learn about essential values and gain a sense of responsibility toward other people in the community. And volunteering does more than teach children to be aware of the needs of others. It also helps them take the focus off their own worries. By giving their time, treasure, and talents to others, children are better able to put their own problems into perspective.

Sadly, many patients I met in my practice were so busy with work commitments that they were reluctant to volunteer to help other people. One of the most common reasons parents gave for not volunteering is that they didn't want to take time away from their families. But did you know that the exact opposite is true? Volunteering with your children actually strengthens your family. You are doing something together that is positive. You gain a shared sense of purpose and mission. In short, sharing a positive and happy volunteer experience is one of the most rewarding activities your family can do.

An increasing number of families are realizing this. Sheryl Nefstead, an associate professor at the University of Minnesota Cooperative Extension Service, identified family volunteerism as an emerging trend in the 1990s. She said, "People are trying to put more emphasis on family cohesiveness, and they're searching for ways to help young people have a sense of hope and satisfaction." In fact, a 1994 Gallup survey reported that more than a third of American households said volunteering together was part of their family life. The most common volunteer activities include helping older people, working

Connect with the Larger Community   217

with youth programs, helping in church or religious programs, assisting in sports or school-related programs, helping in environmental programs, and serving the homeless.

It turns out that giving to others by volunteering is highly healthy for children. It appears to improve their emotional and relational health. Youth who volunteer just one hour a week are 50 percent less likely to abuse drugs, alcohol, cigarettes, or engage in destructive behavior—and they're more likely to do well in school, graduate, vote, and be philanthropic. Children also recognize the benefits of volunteering. Volunteering receives such high marks from teens that they rank it one of the top three activities (along with the environment and eating healthy) that they consider to be "cool." A 1995 Search Institute report found that 55 percent of children who volunteered say it showed them how good it feels to help other people and how much more can be done when people work together as a team.

All the evidence seems to agree: A family volunteer project is one of the most effective ways we can reinforce the important principles of cooperation, teamwork, and respect—all of which are necessary if our children are to successfully interact with the world around them.

Dose of Wisdom

And do not forget to do good and to share with others, for with such sacrifices God is pleased.

Hebrews 13:16, The Bible

TEACHING OUR CHILDREN TO BUILD GREAT FRIENDSHIPS

Teaching our children virtues, such as respect for authority and respect for others, and teaching them the importance of making a positive contribution in the world are essential principles for a highly healthy child and a highly healthy society. But a highly healthy life involves far more than appropriate behavior; it also requires appropriate relationships.

Our children's friends will have, and probably already have had, a huge impact on all aspects of their health. Making friends is one of the first ways children learn to interact with people outside of the family. Through their friendships, children experience for the first time what it means to be part of a larger community. This experience can be either highly healthy or highly unhealthy.

Friends can make the difference between a child being healthy and being lonely and uncomfortable around others. Good friends can offer comfort during tough times and add to the celebration during good times. The benefits of positive friendships show up very early in a child's life. A growing body of research shows that social skills and friendships are as important as academic skills in predicting a child's future health. A child who starts kindergarten and has a friend in his or her class, for example, adjusts better to school than a child who does not start kindergarten with a friend. A child who maintains friendships as the school year progresses likes school better, and those who make new friends in school make greater gains in school performance.

Children who do not have friends or who are repeatedly rejected by their peers can quickly develop what child development experts call "a cycle of rejection." Research shows that children who experience rejection by their peers are more likely to develop serious emotional, relational, and spiritual difficulties later in life. For example, they are more likely to be dissatisfied with themselves and their relationships. They are more likely than other children to experience strong feelings of loneliness and social dissatisfaction, to have lower levels of self-esteem, and to become depressed. If you're tempted to think your child's friends aren't really very important, consider the story a friend of mine shared:

> I still remember being on the school playground in fifth grade. I can see kids bouncing red balls, laughing in small groups. And there I was, alone. I didn't have many friends, and those I did have were also "rejects"—the boy with big ears, the heavy boy. It didn't matter that I was a good student. I was too uncoordinated to do well in sports, and I just didn't fit in with the cliques.

> Did that hurt me? You bet. I tried to reach out sometimes, but when you're always picked on and left out, or are the last one picked for a team, you just want to hide. I became angry and wished I could have friends like most everyone else. I kept wondering what was wrong with me.

> Finally I made what turned out to be a life-changing decision. I watched the kids on the playground and thought, *You think I'm nothing. But that's not true. I'll show you I'm something.* And I lived that way for quite a while, even after I graduated from college with high

honors—still proving to those kids on the school playground that I had worth.

I wish things had been different. I wish I had had more good friends during elementary school and junior high. I wish I had told my parents what was happening. But I didn't know what to do. I certainly didn't know what I now know about the importance of friendships in children's lives. I'm glad I didn't make the opposite choice and think, Okay, you are right. I am worthless. If I had, my life might have gone in a very different direction.

That's powerful, isn't it? Peer rejection is a predictor of later life problems such as dropping out of school, juvenile delinquency, and mental health problems. Dropping out of school is a particularly frequent outcome, with about 25 percent of low-accepted children dropping out of school compared to 8 percent of other children.

Children who don't build friendships seem to have something in common: A large proportion of rejected children lack positive interaction skills, such as being cooperative, helpful, or considerate toward others. My suspicion is that these children have not developed some of the skills and habits we've already discussed. They haven't been trained to "fly" on their own. My belief is that it is not only possible but necessary to teach these children healthier ways to interact with others.

Randy was a hyperactive, energetic, and highly creative five-year-old patient of mine. His mother was concerned about the way he interacted with other children and about his lack of friends. My suspicion was that Randy had never been taught how to interact with others and had parents who lacked these skills as well. So I recommended to Randy's mom that they see a child counselor who I knew would consider the situation from the angle of the family, not just the child. I knew it would be easier for the parents to "take Randy to see the counselor" than to admit that they needed to see the counselor for themselves.

Several months later, Randy's mom came into the office. During the course of our visit, I asked about Randy. She blushed.

"Dr. Larimore," she began, "I'm embarrassed to admit it, but as we got into the counseling, my husband and I realized that Randy's problem was us! We realized that Randy's negative interactions with kids—his unwillingness to cooperate or be helpful with his teachers—was because he hadn't seen positive interactions demonstrated at home."

I smiled on the inside. Randy was another example of a highly unhealthy child who simply needed the teaching, coaching, and training of highly healthy parents.

Obviously we parents can't create or maintain friendships for our children, but we can certainly support and encourage the process. Young children often make friends with children who live in the neighborhood, who attend the same day care center or Sunday school, or who are the children of their parents' friends. So parents of young children should provide sufficient opportunities for their children to meet other children.

As children grow older, the intensity and importance of their friendships change. In elementary school, children tend to pair off by gender—a normal thing to do because boys and girls almost always play differently at this age. They enjoy different games and activities. Boys often play loudly in large groups, while girls form smaller groups around shared activities. At this age, even though our children still rely on us for so much, they are beginning to develop an identity outside the family.

As a parent, you may notice that your "independent" little boy will continue to come inside to get a glass of water or to ask if you saw him do something—or maybe just to ask a question. He's still very much relying on mom and is just checking to be sure she's there and that she cares.

During the later years of elementary school, children begin to develop strong friendships with a particular set of peers. Usually these groups are defined by well-matched personalities—quiet children gathered together, or physically active sports fans forming a group. Sometimes these groups are created by an activity the children share. Children often choose extracurricular activities based on what their friends are doing.

At this stage, your children will rely on you less often and you will need to ask more questions to see how your child is doing. Cleaning-up time before dinner or family discussions at mealtimes can provide great opportunities to ask open-ended questions that encourage children to talk about what they are thinking and doing. You might ask, "What was it like to play with the other children today?" or, "How did you feel when you got an A on your spelling paper?"

If your child has trouble making or finding friends, look for groups or activities at which he or she can feel welcome or can excel. It might be an after-school club for your book lover or a community group for young chess players. Dedicate yourself to helping your child find soul mates who may not be found in your child's normal circle of activities.

Friendship is an area in which parents can make a positive impact on their child for life. Recent medical research has expanded our knowledge of the importance of friendships on our health. We now know that people who do not regularly enjoy meaningful personal relationships with God or others, or who are in relationships devoid of love or caring, are likely to have dramatically lower levels of health. Lonely people are at greater risk for heart attack, heart failure, ulcers, stroke, infectious diseases, mental illness, diabetes, many types of cancer, lung disease, autoimmune disorders, and other life-threatening illnesses. Your child simply cannot be highly healthy without highly healthy friendships!

Resource Box   **Helpful Hints**

Supporting Your Child's Friendships

Although friendships provide necessary forays into the outside world, you are still your child's trainer. Your child still depends on you for direction and support in building these friendships. Here are some tips for supporting and staying connected to your child (adapted from the U.S. Department of Education's "Helping Your Child Through Early Adolescence").

- *Get to know your child's friends.* One way to learn about these friends is to drive them to events. Talking in the car can reveal a lot. Welcome your child's friends into your home. It provides peace of mind, allows you to set the rules of conduct, and helps you gain a better understanding of what is important to them.
- *Get to know the parents of your child's friends.* It helps to know if other parents' attitudes and approaches to parenting are similar to yours. Knowing the other parent makes it easier to learn where your child is going, who else is going along, what time the activity starts and ends, whether an adult will be present, and how your child will get to and from the activity.
- *Help your child learn that friendships based on looks alone are only skin-deep.* One way to help your child choose

the best friends is to help him or her see that good friends have good inner qualities such as loyalty, helpfulness, or a sense of humor. Talk with your child about the qualities of his or her good friends.

- *Provide your child with unstructured time in a safe place to hang around with friends.* Activities are important, but unstructured time with friends in a safe place with adult supervision lets your child share ideas and develop important social skills. For example, when he or she is with friends, your child can learn that good friends are good listeners, that they are helpful and confident (but not overly so), that they are enthusiastic, that they possess a sense of humor, and that they respect others. Spending time with others may also help your child change some behaviors that make others uncomfortable around him or her—being too serious or unenthusiastic, too critical of others, or too stubborn.

TEACHING OUR CHILDREN TO SEEK OUT MENTORS

As parents, we're not responsible for providing our children with *all* of the assets and skills they need to succeed in the world they are inheriting from us. Our children will have needs, talents, gifts, and interests that are beyond ours, so we must be willing to link our children to programs and people who can help fulfill their needs. This is where mentors come in. Mentors can include extended family members, teachers, coaches, youth pastors, camp counselors, Sunday school teachers, Scout leaders, and many others.

Not only do our children's friends have an impact on their transition into adulthood, the positive mentors who spend time with our children also play a crucial role in their transition from childhood to adulthood. The mentoring process is critical to the healthy development of children. It can help children to be happy, healthy, and wise. In fact, the research suggests that the sharing of unconditional positive regard of one person for another is one major impact of a child's positive mentors. We parents must understand that our children's transition from dependence on us to healthy relationships with positive mentors is a highly healthy process. Let me share a personal example.

Bill Judge has been a dairy farmer for the better part of seven decades. He knows a lot about cattle and is a member of the Florida Cattle Breeders Hall of Fame. He has been involved in international mission organizations, has served as an elder in his church, and has raised five beautiful daughters. But to me, Bill, above all else, is my mentor. For sixteen years, we met almost every Tuesday morning at Joanie's Diner in Kissimmee, Florida. Bill held me accountable to be a good family physician, a good husband, and a good father. He helped me in my spiritual disciplines and is one of my best friends.

Bill gave me another very important gift by being a mentor for my son, Scott. Bill would call to talk with Scott and always made his home open to him. Scott, in turn, could call Mr. Judge or go over to his home any time— night or day. After we moved to Colorado Springs, Scott went back to Kissimmee to serve as a substitute teacher at the high school from which he had graduated. During that season of his life, he chose to call Mr. Judge and asked if they could meet weekly in a formal mentoring relationship.

Adult role models outside the home can either supplement or detract from your work as a parent. In Bill's case, he enhanced my role as a dad. Scott was able to "check things out with Mr. Bill." When Scott learned that Bill backed up what I was teaching and saying—and in many areas felt even more strongly than I—Scott's trust in me grew. In addition, Scott could talk with Bill about things he might not feel comfortable sharing with Barb or me.

Resource Box   Helpful Hints

Mentors and Their Positive Impact on Children

Let's look at some of the positive ways in which mentors influence children (adapted from mentoring facts provided by the Wise Men and Women Mentorship Program):

- Mentors make children feel unique, special, and good about themselves.
- Mentors provide children with consistent and unconditional support, which helps children feel safe in their world.
- Mentors allow children to become attached to them, which increases the child's ability to form nurturing relationships with others.

- Mentors model positive values, attitudes, and behaviors, which encourages children to do likewise.
- Mentors help children discover solutions to their problems, which increases their sense of confidence and self-reliance.
- Mentors help children look beyond today and to see tomorrow's possibilities, which increases their sense of hope and raises their expectations for the future.

We are just beginning to realize how important mentors are in the lives of children. The results of the first national study of mentoring proved that positive mentoring virtually always enriches young people's lives. Youth who met regularly with a mentor were 46 percent less likely to begin using illegal drugs, 52 percent less likely to skip school, and 33 percent less likely to get into fights. Students who had relationships with positive mentors reported greater confidence in their performance at school and better relationships with their parents and siblings.

Positive mentors for children can enhance the character traits we parents work so hard to foster in our children: self-esteem, a sense of hope, a sense of safety, positive relationships, positive social orientation, and high self-expectations. These character traits help protect children from negative risk factors such as poverty, unemployment, substance abuse, marital conflict, gangs, and social violence. Positive mentors can help us prevent unhealthy outcomes in our children's lives, help them cope better with adversity, and serve as role models and guides on our children's pathway toward adulthood. In the recipe of helping children become highly healthy adults, positive mentors are important ingredients.

Let me add a note of caution here. Parents need to be as selective in their choice of a mentor as they are in choosing other adults who interact with their children. Some men and women are child predators—though it's much more common in men. Homosexual activists would have us believe there's no connection between homosexuality and the sexual abuse of children, but the evidence I've reviewed leads me to believe that a significant number of gay men seek out adolescent males or young boys as sexual partners, and some have been known to seek their victims via mentoring programs.

Most mentors, however, are good and honorable people. Most of us can recall individuals who positively influenced our development, even if we knew them for only a short time. Most of us remember the adults who touched our lives in a positive way—someone who was a wise and trusted friend and guide. While I was writing this chapter, I received the email journal of Senator John Andrews, president of the Colorado Senate, who wrote these poignant words about a few of his mentors:

> The experiences that imprinted me deeply before I was 20, the places and especially the people, seem more treasured as I near 60.... Those days and those faces are always with me, bittersweet in some ways, yet beloved.... Here is a roll call of unforgettables from just beyond the family circle, some of the many who will be held in my heart for as long as it beats.
>
> Lucille Perrill, my first-grade teacher, taught me about high expectations. Bill Van Vleck, a golf and tennis buddy of my dad's, modeled male friendship for my brother and me.... Zoe Wasson, a leader in our church, shines as an emblem of holiness in my boyhood memories....
>
> Gillian Elliott, an English import, magically awakened my love of literature in the sixth grade....
>
> Mary Kessler ... [became] my chief encourager in reading and writing, succeeded the year after that by Irma Eareckson. There was something wonderfully timeless in knowing that Miss Eareckson, like Miss Perrill, had also taught my father.

Teaching our children the skills they need to be able to invest in the world around them and fostering their interactions within that world are essential to their well-being. By doing this in such a way that we slowly and responsibly lengthen the tether, we will set our children free to soar into the world in a way that improves the health of the family and community into which they land. As Senator Andrews has wisely pointed out, "Who we each are is largely a product of who we've shared our lives with, especially the early chapters. May we never cease to hold those people tight."

Chapter Ten

Instill a Balanced Self-Concept

Not long after we moved to Bryson City, North Carolina, a Smoky Mountain hamlet of about a thousand citizens and more than thirty churches, we began attending a church that had Wednesday evening fellowship suppers. Attending these dinners enabled us to get to know many people, and the food was beyond compare. We usually brought Kate, and she sat in a high chair between us. She was just under three years old, and cerebral palsy had slowed her development so she was just learning to talk.

One night we sat across the table from Joe and Peggy Ashley. Joe was a ranger for the Great Smoky Mountains National Park, and Peggy was a nurse at our hospital. As we introduced ourselves, Peggy looked across the table at Kate, who was devouring her meal, and asked, "Well, young lady, what is your name?"

Kate looked up at her and, without hesitation, replied, "Good Girl."

Peggy looked flustered. "What?"

Kate cocked her head to the side, smiled, and repeated, "Good Girl."

Barb and I were stunned. "Her name's Kate," Barb answered, to clear up the confusion. We all chuckled nervously.

Later that night, Barb thought aloud, "It must be from all the encouragement we give her. When she stands or rolls over, it's such a great accomplishment that either you or I always exclaim, 'Good girl!' She must think that's her name!"

We smiled at the implications. "Good Girl Larimore," Barb sighed. "It does have a nice ring to it." I laughed. It did.

This was an important lesson for us as young parents to learn. Through our spoken words, we were giving Kate a concept of who she was. Even at her early age, she had come to believe that her efforts to walk and talk were good and, even more important, that *she* was good! Thus, a positive self-image was begun.

Child development experts tell us that when a child believes he or she is a certain kind of person, that belief guides his or her behavior. This truth has powerful implications in the lives of children. Let me illustrate. During elementary school, Kate concluded that she was not social. Because of her delayed language skills and hyperacute listening skills, she wouldn't initiate conversations with her classmates. She thought, *Since I don't talk very well, how can I talk to people?* When she didn't initiate talking, her classmates felt she wasn't interested in socializing and wouldn't talk with her. When Kate saw that others apparently didn't like talking to her, it confirmed her belief that she was not social.

When Barb and I discovered what was happening, we taught Kate how to start conversations with her classmates. Before long, she had several new friends. She continued to practice her social and language skills, and many of the friendships started then continue today.

In contrast, consider Lee. His mother found it difficult to love anyone. By the time Lee was born, she had been married three times. Her second husband had divorced her because *she* beat him up regularly. Lee's mom gave him no affection, no love, no discipline, and no training during his early years, so his concept of self was shipwrecked very early in life. No one helped Lee develop a healthier view of himself. In fact, when Lee was thirteen, a school psychologist commented that he probably didn't even know the meaning of the word *love*.

Despite his high IQ, Lee failed academically and dropped out of high school. The Marine Corps reportedly built men, and Lee wanted to be one—so he signed up. But his childhood self-concept went with him. Lee eventually was court-martialed and thrown out of the Corps.

In his early twenties, Lee was friendless and stranded. He had a terrible self-concept and no sense of worth. He tried to make it on his own but failed in marriage and at work. Finally, he took a rifle from his garage and carried it to his newly acquired job at a book-storage company. From a window on the sixth floor, shortly after noon on November 22, 1963, he sent two bullets crashing into the head of President John Fitzgerald Kennedy.

Lee Harvey Oswald, the rejected and unloved failure, killed the man who perhaps more than any other man at the time embodied the success, beauty, wealth, and family affection Lee lacked. I'm not saying that Lee's parental rejection and personal problems excuse or justify his behavior. But no one could describe him as having had a healthy childhood or a healthy self-concept. He illustrates the sad truth that children whose sense of self is either falsely deflated or overly inflated face a high risk of never becoming highly healthy.

I've cared for scores of patients who suffered from physical, emotional, relational, or spiritual pain resulting from a diseased image of themselves. Mark, for example, was brought to my office because his teacher said he was hyperactive. In his case, poor school performance and high distractibility were not due to ADHD. Mark suffered from a severe lack of self-confidence, which often results in a wide variety of unhealthy behaviors and attitudes. Although Mark's symptoms were similar to those of ADHD, the treatment was vastly different.

Children who lack confidence tend to focus on failure instead of success, problems instead of challenges, and difficulties instead of possibilities. As a result, they can become distractible, disruptive, driven, and demanding, or—on the other end of the spectrum—shy, withdrawn, passive, and dependent. A lack of confidence is simply one manifestation of a damaged self-concept.

WHAT CAUSES A CHILD'S CONCEPT OF SELF TO BECOME UNBALANCED?

Counselors and psychologists tell me that in virtually every case, an unhealthy self-concept originates during childhood. Parents, teachers, and peers are very important influences on a developing child's self-concept. Let's explore the impact of each.

The Influence of Parents

A mother and a father are designed and destined to have an intense and lasting influence on their children. Their voices of encouragement and praise are the first and most influential voices their children hear. Not surprisingly, children are most highly healthy when they are nurtured and deeply cared for by a loving, sensitive, committed, and married mom and dad.

When children sense their parents' pleasure with their first steps or first words, they smile and want more affirmation. So parents who praise their children for success are more likely to see success. As parents encourage their children to try new things and to develop their talents, gifts, and abilities, their children develop a healthy sense of pride in their accomplishments. Regardless of wealth, health, or circumstances, children who receive this type of parenting from a mother and a father are more likely to grow up feeling loved, valued, and significant. They are more likely to have healthy, happy feelings about themselves.

It's easy to see how this kind of encouragement and affirmation contributes to a child's self-concept. But parental influence on a child's self-concept goes even deeper; it influences the very foundation of a child's self-image. My daughter, Kate, shares a precious friendship with John and Stasi Eldredge, and through Kate I've come to know John, who is trained as a counselor and is now a well-known author. At a retreat deep in the Rocky Mountains, John shared with me his belief about the formation of self-image in children. I think his insights are crucial to understanding our role as parents, so I want to share them with you.

Eldredge believes every boy wants to know, *Am I strong? Am I a true man? Do I have what it takes?* These questions *must* be answered by his dad. Every girl wants to know, *Am I beautiful? Am I worthy of rescue?* These questions *must* be answered primarily by her father. According to Eldredge, boy and girls (and, when they grow up, men and women) seek the answer to these most basic of questions from childhood until death. The answers they receive, especially from their fathers, either build the foundation for an incredibly powerful and positive self-image or severely wound that image—resulting in what Eldredge calls "the false self."

What's interesting to me is that, as children are admired by and believed in by their parents, they develop value, significance, and confidence, which almost always comes to expression in good feelings toward others. There is a beautifully designed cycle at work here. Children who are loved, encouraged, and affirmed feel confident, and they feel good about themselves. As a result, they are secure and caring enough to love and affirm others.

Sadly, some parents don't provide this type of care and affirmation. Imagine the devastating impact of a father who says to his son, "You're just a momma's boy," or says to his daughter, "You're not pretty enough for anybody." These verbal blows are like a knife thrust into the heart. Furthermore, words of affirmation that go unspoken, affection that is withheld, and cheerleading that is not given can be just as destructive. These wounds deposit a deep uncertainty in the soul, leaving a wounded and broken heart that will influence the child's physical, emotional, relational, and spiritual health for life.

Samantha, a former patient, stands out as a painful reminder of this truth. She could *never* do anything right in her father's eyes. Samantha's father didn't dispense love; he meted out the law and doled out severe punishment for any perceived infraction. Her dad always was critical of her—never encouraging or loving. One time she told me, with tears in her eyes, "He's never even hugged me." He communicated to her clearly, *You are not lovely. You are not worthy.*

It's no surprise that Samantha grew up without a healthy self-concept. As she entered her teenage years, she didn't believe she could accomplish anything of value. She lacked a sense of self-worth or self-confidence. She sought other men to show her she was worthy. They only used her. Through the years she's made some terrible decisions and is, as of this writing, a terribly unhealthy young woman.

Countless children are raised in homes where the kind of negative parenting Samantha experienced occurs. Harmful, unconstructive comments and cruel, merciless criticism are fed into the psyche of these children daily until their spirits are broken. Day by day their confidence is stripped away and replaced with hesitation, indecision, and uncertainty. They are horribly wounded.

Resource Box **Helpful Hints**

We parents often fail to realize the powerful influence we have in shaping our children's self-concept. It's so easy to kill a child's confidence and crush their hearts by what we say or do. Here are a few confidence-killers I'm sure you'll want to avoid:

- failing to recognize the difference between childish irresponsibility and defiant behavior
- administering punishment or discipline in anger
- being unnecessarily overprotective or anxious
- giving overbearing, harsh, or unnecessary criticism
- failing to encourage or praise
- making mean-spirited or unflattering comparisons to siblings or friends
- having unrealistic or age-inappropriate expectations
- pushing for unnecessary or excessive competition

You must be there for your child. You must continually answer his or her most basic questions.

The Influence of Teachers

Many, if not most, teachers are skilled, nurturing, and helpful mentors for children. They know how to help children learn. They know how to build self-esteem and self-confidence. They know how to recognize learning styles and temperaments. When teamed with nurturing parents, teachers can be a child's most helpful guides in developing a positive view of self.

However, one bad apple can ruin the whole bushel! A poor teacher can undermine a child's concept of self. I saw this in Derek, a patient I delivered and saw for a number of years. In the office, he was very quiet. He seemed shy and withdrawn, but once I learned how to talk to him, he became very conversational. He was intelligent and got along well with his brothers and sister, but his parents had a difficult marriage, and life at home was tense. Derek's dad was a strict, violent disciplinarian and, I was told, always criticized Derek for being stupid.

One teacher after another scolded Derek for daydreaming at school. He was criticized in front of classmates for not listening. His performance suffered; his confidence plummeted. His teachers never realized that Derek was simply escaping to another world because his world at home was so painful. Because they missed this fact, they compounded the problem by their disparagement, ridicule, and condemnation.

When he was ten years old, Derek attempted suicide and was admitted to a psychiatric hospital. A caring psychiatrist, a psychological care team, and I were able to unravel Derek's destructive past. The psychiatrist pointed out that occasional negative experiences with a parent or friend or teacher are not usually harmful, but that in Derek's case, the constant, unremitting criticism and mockery by his teachers—who other than his mom were his only potentially positive role models and mentors—combined with his very sensitive, vulnerable nature to result in a broken child.

Thankfully, we were able to get Derek's parents into a parenting-skills class. Derek's dad learned how to affirm Derek's masculinity, and they began to spend time together. His principal worked to ensure that his teachers were skilled and nurturing. Derek's youth pastor and youth group came alongside to support him as well. As a result, this broken boy is developing into a healthy young adult. He's currently in college, and his concept of self seems well on the way to becoming well-balanced.

The Influence of Friends, Playmates, and Classmates

There's no doubt that parents have by far the greatest influence—for good or bad—on their children because of the time they do—or don't—spend together and because of the emotional connection between them. But many other voices tell children they are or are not valued, that they are or are not normal; many try to convince them who they should be. It may be hard to believe, but a child's friends, playmates, and classmates may be the second most influential cause of an unbalanced concept of self. Children can be very mean-spirited toward one another, and their actions can do heartbreaking damage.

Who among us, as we think back to our childhood years, didn't at one time or another feel different, awkward, or weird? At some time, virtually all children feel senselessly inferior. Rather than appreciating their uniqueness, they tend to "compare and despair." They tend to believe that not being like everyone else is a problem they must solve by conforming. The pressure to conform is so great that children who dare to be authentic and different are often ostracized, bullied, ridiculed, and forsaken.

Girls may be the worst culprits. They can often be incredibly jealous, critical, and rejecting. As a girl tries to establish her own value and worth to others, she may criticize, exclude, and ridicule other girls. Girls can make it very unpleasant for girls they don't consider to be worthy of their "inner circle."

Competition among children, whether it is about possessions, sports, looks, hairstyle, clothes, friends, or grades, is universal. There is no way any child will excel in every area. Some children will fall out of the norm in some areas, and some in most areas. When compared only to the very best students, for example, perfectly average students may feel inferior. So it's very easy for children to believe they are unable to measure up to what they perceive to be normal.

Unnecessary comparisons and improperly administered criticism can leave children with impressions or mental imprints they carry the rest of their lives. These internally programmed messages can become loud, raucous, and negative self-talk, causing a child to think, *I can't do it well enough, so I won't even try!* or, *Others always do it better, no matter how hard I try, so I may as well just give up right now.* A boy may wonder, *Am I really a man? Do I really have what it takes?* A girl may wonder, *Am I really lovely?* These false beliefs not only cause a false or unbalanced view of self, they can derail or destroy self-confidence unless someone—hopefully parents—counters the potentially toxic impact children can have on children. A mom and a dad are a potent antidote against this poison to a child's heart.

How Do Children Handle Inferiority?

Psychiatrist Paul Meier uses the acronym A-C-T-I-O-N to describe common ways children handle feelings of inferiority. Perhaps you will recognize your child's tendencies in this list:

A = Alike-ism: I can hide myself by being like everyone else. I must not be different in appearance and behavior.

C = Compensation: I'll find what I can do well and concentrate on it. That way I'll be accepted and respected for something.

T = Trip out: It's impossible to make the pain go away, so I will hide in activities or drugs and alcohol.

I = Introversion: If I'm quiet, maybe no one will know I exist. If I open my mouth or take initiative, I might make a mistake and people would laugh at me.

O = Obstinate: I will pretend I'm tough and crude. I can bluff people into thinking I'm confident by the way I show disrespect to others.

N = Nitwitty: I will be a clown. I'll do stupid things to make people laugh, especially at me. I won't believe they're laughing at me for any reason other than because I make them laugh. I feel important when I make people happy.

ESTABLISHING A FOUNDATION FOR YOUR CHILD'S SELF-CONCEPT

The evidence gathered from many studies shows that parents who instill a positive sense of self in their children will have children who reap long-term benefits in physical and mental health, educational achievement, and social and emotional functioning. Positive early life experiences contribute to socio-economic and physical health measures, improved well-being, and improved responses to stressful circumstances. So helping your children feel good about themselves—tending to their sense of self and their self-confidence—is one of the greatest responsibilities and biggest challenges you have as a parent. The foundation you help build has a dramatic impact on each of their health wheels.

Children who have a positive sense of self feel a sense of internal worth. They feel they have something worthwhile to contribute, so they are able to venture out into the world, work toward attaining their goals, and tend to welcome life with anticipation and pleasure. Other benefits of a healthy, balanced concept of self include the following:

- greater social health, including sexual identity and behavior
- an ability to resist premature sex and unhealthy relationships
- a capacity to love and to receive love
- an ability to welcome challenges and work cooperatively with others
- greater intellectual health
- appropriate and balanced beliefs about their abilities and what they are willing to tackle
- greater physical health, which diminishes the tendency toward high-risk (and potentially fatal) behaviors such as drugs, some extreme sports, fringe behaviors, and sexual risks
- a tendency to become spiritually healthy

In short, a healthy self-concept results in highly healthy children who know they are loved and know they are valuable—to their parents, their family, their community, and their God.

With these benefits in mind, let's explore some of the principles you as a parent can follow to help put in place the foundation your children need to develop a balanced, healthy self-concept. I know you want to do the very best job you can. If you (or your spouse, if you are married) were not raised in a home that nurtured a balanced concept of self, now is the time to break this cycle. Even if you were blessed to have been raised in a nurturing home, these principles can serve as a mirror for identifying areas in which you can improve your parenting skills and effectiveness.

Build on the Right Foundation

I believe the principles for a healthy concept of self are found in the wisdom of the Bible. If this wisdom is understood and owned by the child, it has the potential to form a self-concept on which a child can build for a lifetime. If a child realizes at an early age that he or she was created and gifted by God and is loved by God, these truths will be life-changing.

According to the Bible, every person—every child—is designed by our Creator to be unique. We are *not* to be like anyone else. No other person in history has had or ever will have the same set of genes, the same fingerprints, the same brain waves, and the exact same life-experiences and perspectives as your child. Let me share a poem written by David, one of the greatest kings of ancient Israel. He eloquently describes God's hand in creating each child:

> *O Lord, you have searched me*
> > *and you know me.*
> *You know when I sit and when I rise;*
> > *you perceive my thoughts from afar.*
> *You discern my going out and my lying down;*
> > *you are familiar with all my ways.*
> *Before a word is on my tongue*
> > *you know it completely, O Lord.*
>
> *You hem me in—behind and before;*
> > *you have laid your hand upon me.*
> *Such knowledge is too wonderful for me,*
> > *too lofty for me to attain.*
>
> *Where can I go from your Spirit?*
> > *Where can I flee from your presence?...*
>
> *For you created my inmost being;*
> > *you knit me together in my mother's womb.*
> *I praise you because I am fearfully and wonderfully made;*
> > *your works are wonderful,*
> > *I know that full well.*
> *My frame was not hidden from you*
> > *when I was made in the secret place.*
> *When I was woven together in the depths of the earth,*
> > *your eyes saw my unformed body.*
> *All the days ordained for me*
> > *were written in your book*
> > *before one of them came to be.*

What a beautiful piece of wisdom this is! Can you imagine how sharing this view could cause a child's self-concept and self-esteem to grow and flower? Can you imagine how teaching this to your children could cause them to see themselves as their Creator sees them?

The three most basic spiritual and emotional human needs are a positive relationship with God, a positive relationship with oneself, and positive relationships with others. If a boy hates or dislikes himself, has no self-confidence or no realistic view of who he has been created to be, how can this boy truly love others? How can a girl love herself in a healthy way unless she is bolstered by the knowledge that she is deeply loved by the God who designed and created her? The first key to building a healthy concept of self is for children to learn how God views them.

Even if you haven't placed much stock in the Bible's wisdom in the past, I encourage you to help your children understand their value in God's sight. It is imperative that our children learn that their worth and value do *not* come from accomplishments, physical attributes, intelligence, or possessions. True worth comes from the value that their Creator gives them and from the destiny he intends them to fulfill.

A child's relationship with God can reprogram the damaging influence of others. A child who is taught and then internalizes the truth that he or she is created in God's image and is a masterpiece designed by him cannot help but be affirmed. What greater source of confidence can there be for our children than knowing that the Creator of the universe is acquainted with each of them personally? What greater sense of worth could our children have other than that which results from the Creator of the universe valuing them highly? What could be more highly healthy than for our children to grow to understand that God knows and understands each one of our fears and worries? What greater comfort can we give our children than teaching them that the loving God is reaching out to them and has an immeasurable love for them—even if other people don't seem to care for and about them? Imagine their confidence when they come to understand that only God can turn their liabilities, mistakes, and wrongdoing into assets. Only he can convert their inevitable feelings of emptiness into fullness.

This is self-worth and self-confidence at their most appropriate and richest levels. This is not a self-worth and self-confidence that is dependent on the whims of birth, social placement, or material goods. When applied to life, this foundation encourages a child to seek out his or her destiny and look for God-directed opportunities as opposed to wilting in a poor self-image or running amok with an overinflated self-image. Only a healthy relationship with God can free our children (and us) from the tyranny of a deflated or an overinflated self. Without question, the most valuable contribution we parents can make to our children is to guide them toward a genuine and personal relationship with their Creator.

The second key to a highly healthy self-concept is the presence of a father and mother who positively and constructively answer the child's basic questions I discussed earlier.

Although we've been focusing our attention on the risks of a poor self-concept, I must interject a few words of caution regarding the opposite problem—an overinflated self-concept. We see the danger in allowing our children to view themselves as having less value than their Creator has given to them, but it's equally dangerous for them to be arrogant and self-important.

I bring this up because, in the absence of wisdom from the Bible, some child experts, psychologists, and teachers promote inappropriate pride under the guise of self-esteem or self-confidence. In an effort to counter negative influences that tear down self-confidence, they encourage children to be selfish, do their own thing, search for self-fulfillment, and look out for number one. They wrongly teach children, "You can do anything you want to do!" However, nothing is further from the truth.

I think of David, a young man I met at a camp. He dreamed of being an NBA or NFL star, but he wasn't very skilled in sports. Yet he told me, "If you dream it, you can do it!" But in David's case, he could dream about being a professional athlete until the cows came home. He didn't need a sports agent; he needed a dose of reality. He needed adults—parents, teachers, counselors—who cared for him enough to help him align his dreams and hopes with his God-given gifts and help him discover *his* destiny.

Benny also illustrates what can happen when a child believes that he or she can do or be anything. He wanted to be a doctor, just like his dad. His parents weren't pushing him to be a doctor. In fact, Benny's mom told me, "Dr. Walt, I believe God has created him for another purpose. Benny isn't gifted in the sciences. But he's great at relationships, especially with kids. I wonder if he's not best suited to be a teacher or coach, maybe a camp counselor or youth pastor."

One of Benny's key mentors during middle school and high school had bought into the myth that any child can grow up to be *anything* he or she wants to be. "If you just work hard enough at your dreams, Benny," this misguided mentor would exhort, "you can become what you dream." So when Benny went to college, he started out in premed and promptly flunked out.

All was not lost, however. Benny began listening to his mom and dad. He took advantage of testing and counseling provided by his college. It was no surprise to his parents when he tested at the top for those gifted to go into communications. Benny changed his major and is now at the top of his class. I'm not sure where he'll end up, but his picture of himself is more accurate and healthy than it was. He seems headed now toward a much more successful, confident, and significant life.

Love Each Child Unconditionally

Love is the first and most basic of all emotional needs. When children are loved in a healthy way, they feel that they belong and that they have value and significance. A child who is loved knows that his or her feelings, thoughts, and opinions matter. Children who know they are loved by God, their parents, and significant others are much more likely to become highly healthy.

But not all love is equal. Parents typically use one of two different kinds of love: *conditional love,* which is highly unhealthy, and *unconditional love,* which is highly healthy. Most parents use both kinds of love at one time or another, but they lean toward using one type more often. Highly healthy parents strive to habitually express unconditional love.

Conditional love is an earned love. It requires certain behaviors and approved actions. If you love your children only if they perform well, or because they behave well, you are expressing conditional love—and it's not healthy. *But,* you may be thinking, *what's wrong with that? Shouldn't I expect my children to obey and to do their best?* Of course! You shouldn't accept willfully defiant and inappropriate behavior. However, even when the behavior is unacceptable, you should *always* love the child.

Unconditional love means that you love your children no matter what. It doesn't matter how much or how little ability, physical beauty, personality, or brains your child possesses. It doesn't matter how well your child behaves. *Unconditional love is always there.*

Unconditional love is the ideal for which parents should continually strive. Only unconditional love enables us to meet our children's most basic emotional, relational, and spiritual needs. Only with a nurturing foundation of unconditional love can parents find the balance between being too harsh and too lenient. Unconditional love, when mixed with honest recognition and praise, is a vital ingredient in nurturing a highly healthy child. Will we hit this mark 100 percent of the time? Of course not! Although Barb and I have worked to love unconditionally, all too often we have failed.

Remember when I wrote about Kate calling herself "Good Girl"? Barb and I hadn't communicated the right kind of love to her. We wanted Kate, even with her significant physical disabilities, to develop a balanced self-image and a healthy self-confidence. So we praised and encouraged her, but our praises led her to believe that her value was based on performance. The truth is, we loved her regardless of whether she walked or talked. It would have been better for us to say, "Good job," "Well done," or "I'm so pleased with how hard you're trying." These would have been comments on her performance, not statements of her value.

Children should always be loved for who they are, not for what they do. By now I'm sure you realize that loving our children unconditionally is a skill we learn. Unconditional love starts simply by making a cognitive and deliberate choice. Literally, unconditional love means loving with your head and trusting your heart to follow. So let's explore the steps we can take to learn to love unconditionally.

Seek to Understand Your Child's Temperament

Each child has distinct, recognizable patterns of behavior that are apparent from birth. By understanding your child's temperament, you are better equipped to put your child's behavior in perspective and then to know how to express love for your child. Although various experts describe a child's temperament in different ways, I found it beneficial to teach the parents of my young patients to think in terms of the three basic temperament styles described by Drs. Herbert Birch, Stella Chess, and Alexander Thomas:

- *Pliable or flexible children.* These children are the easiest to raise. They are easygoing. They easily adapt to circumstances and tend to be compliant. If this type of child is your first child, you will think you are a brilliant parent.
- *Hard or rigid children.* These children—called "strong-willed" by Dr. James Dobson—require the most parenting skill and energy. Their moods can change quickly. They tend to adapt slowly to change. They can be more negative and less compliant than other children. When given boundaries, these children will lean against them—if not rapidly cross them.

- *Slow-to-warm-up children.* These children adapt slowly but tend to be more obedient and compliant than rigid children. Their moods vary, but they do so more slowly than those of rigid children. These children require you to be patient and clear in communicating expectations.

Of course, some children don't fit clearly into one category. Nevertheless, these categories provide a starting point for understanding your children and learning how to express unconditional love for them.

We parents need to understand our own temperaments as well because they influence how we feel about our children. For example, if you are more laid-back and less intense, a slow-to-warm-up or pliable child will be much easier for you to parent. You may find it more difficult to keep a rigid child's behavior from determining the way you express your love for the child. However, if you are energetic, full of life, and always on the go, you may perceive a pliable child to be dull or dreary.

Provide Plenty of Focused Attention

Much of the parental communication directed toward a child is task-oriented: "Have you finished your homework?" "Did you take out the trash?" Communication from a child to a parent often occurs when parents are doing something else, such as reading the newspaper or watching television. So it's crucial for parents to learn to give focused attention when their child is communicating. Focused attention means looking into the eyes of the child and listening and speaking exclusively to the child—which is especially important for men to understand, since they typically focus on only one stimulus at a time. A dad will need to put down the newspaper or turn off the TV to focus on his child. Focused attention from a parent sends a strong message to the child: *I value you, and what you have to say is important to me.*

Give Plenty of Appropriate Physical Contact

Parents can genuinely touch their youngster's heart through appropriate touch. Appropriate touch can be a light back massage, a toss of her hair, a friendly pat on the shoulder, a hug, or a hand or foot massage. Although it may seem insignificant, the use of touch by parents sends a powerful message to their children, particularly teenagers. Touch communicates, *You are important to me and worthy of my interest and my time.*

Appreciate the Uniqueness of Each Child

Parents can effectively communicate unconditional love by appreciating the uniqueness of a child, even if the child has little in common with other family members. Children aren't clones of mom or dad—a fact that seems to trouble some parents. While it's quite possible to have a child with whom you have little in common, it doesn't make one of you right and the other wrong; it simply means you're different.

Don't assign importance to only those attributes you hold dear, such as being thin, playing a particular sport, or being mechanical. Instead, help each child recognize his or her uniqueness. Here's a suggestion I offer to help parents accept their child's uniqueness and preferences for activities: An attribute or an activity is just a different choice, not a wrong choice, if you can answer no to the following:

- Is it illegal?
- Is it immoral?
- Is it going to make a difference in five years?
- Is it something that will hurt someone?
- Is it inappropriate for his or her age level?

Don't Allow Your Ego to Get Wrapped Up in the Child

When children are born, parents quickly count fingers and toes and are delighted when everything is normal. From that point on, however, some parents are never satisfied again because their ego is wrapped up in the child's accomplishments. They long for the exceptional child who amazes and dazzles the world. They become addicted to the strokes they get from their child's successes. But no child should have to bear the responsibility for a parent's feelings of self-worth. We must develop a good self-image apart from our children—and allow our children to follow their own destiny.

Encourage Your Child's Belief in Himself or Herself

Parents should do whatever is necessary to encourage their child's belief in himself or herself. As parents, we are like mirrors to our children. Our children will see themselves as we see them. Never see a child as a problem. Make sure that what your child sees in your eyes is positive and affirming.

NURTURING YOUR CHILD'S SELF-CONCEPT

A foundation of unconditional love is the crucial first step for a child to develop a healthy self-concept. When children feel loved, they want to do their best. Parents can nurture or kill this desire by the way they interact with their children on a daily basis. Let's explore several ways parents can foster healthy interaction that will build on a foundation of unconditional love.

Understand and Use the Appropriate Love Languages with Your Children

In their book *The Five Love Languages of Children,* Gary Chapman and Ross Campbell propose that children primarily express and receive love through one of the following communication styles, or "love languages": words of affirmation, acts of service, quality time, physical touch, and receiving gifts. Chapman and Campbell also believe, as I do, that we parents must learn to speak our children's love languages in order to help them balance their concept of self. They write, "Moms and dads can use this information to help them meet their children's deepest emotional needs." Because love language is so important to our ability to express unconditional love, I'll highlight characteristics of each one so you can think about ways to better communicate love to your child. As you read, see if you can pick out the love language of each of your children:

Words of Affirmation

Verbal compliments and words of appreciation can powerfully communicate love. They are best expressed in simple, straightforward affirmations such as, "What a nice dress!" or, "I appreciate that you took out the trash without my even having to ask," or, "The art project you brought home from school is beautiful."

Children who speak the "words of affirmation" love language need to hear truthful words of encouragement and praise constantly. They know they are loved when their parents affirm them with loving words. However, words (even "positive" comments) spoken with a nasty or harsh tone of voice are extremely harmful. Negative words cut more deeply into the spirit of a child who speaks the "words of affirmation" love language, so correction should be done very carefully.

GOD'S DESIGN *for the* HIGHLY HEALTHY CHILD

Acts of Service

These children don't need to be *told* they are loved nearly as much as they need you to *show* them you love them. They need to see love in action. They respond to special meals or packed lunches. They are elated when they get to go on a special outing or shopping trip with you. If you bake a cake or cookies, you win this child's affection.

A word of caution: If you are a "words of affirmation" parent, you may become unhappy if your child doesn't express his or her love verbally. An "acts of service" child may never verbally express love to Mom or Dad but may do small things for them instead. The parent who misses the significance of these little acts misses wonderful opportunities to accept and return the child's love.

If you think your "acts of service" child doesn't love you, and you stop doing the special things that demonstrate love to your child, your child will become unhappy. Why? He or she doesn't *see* you saying, "I love you." Do you see how easily a negative cycle can begin—and why it's important to know the love languages you and your children use?

Quality Time

Children who use the "quality time" love language feel most loved when their parents spend time with *them,* and them alone. This means you give your *undivided* attention to your child—not to them and to television, paying bills, or reading the newspaper. When you devote all your attention to the child—talking with him or her, or just being together—he or she feels loved.

A quick "Hey, how was your day?" or "Better get ready for bed!" will not be adequate for quality-timers. They need to talk to you about their day *and* about how they feel about the day *and* about how you feel about their day. Then they want to know about your day *and* about how you feel about your day, *and* then they'll tell you how they feel about your day. Are you getting the picture? "Quality time" children crave your time and attention, and they need it often. If they don't get it, they'll believe you don't love them all that much—no matter what you say, do, or give them.

Physical Touch

All children (and adults!) need to be touched. Babies left alone in orphanage cribs have died because no one held them, touched them, and cooed to them. Touching is therapeutic. Children whose love language is "physical touch" especially need gentle, loving touches. They crave hugs, a hand on the shoulder, holding hands, a kiss on the cheek, a pat on the back, running your fingers through their hair. If a highly healthy person needs eight hugs a day, multiply it by four if you have a "physical touch" child!

Receiving Gifts

Virtually all of us give our children gifts at holiday times and on their birthdays. Children are usually happy to receive gifts, but if your child rides high for days, weeks, or months because you gave him or her a special gift, chances are you have a "receiving gifts" child.

"Receiving gifts" children are not greedier than other children; they simply need parents who give them things as an expression of their love. Small, thoughtful gifts—the candy bar, the special hair ribbon, the sports team souvenir—make "receiving gifts" children feel loved. Parents don't have to break the bank to help these children feel loved, but they need to be creative and spontaneous about giving small tokens of affection often.

You may be wondering, *Don't all children need to receive love in all of these languages?* My answer is yes! However, each particular child needs to receive love primarily in *one* of these languages. Parents can almost always recognize their primary love language and those of their children. Then it's up to each parent to use the appropriate language.

Recognize the Power of Your Words

The words we speak and the tone of voice we use are extremely powerful. What we say can build up and strengthen our child's concept of self, or it can throw it off balance and perhaps destroy it. Many times we aren't aware of the impact of the words we speak in haste, in anger, or in elevated tones. In my office, in the church lobby, or in the supermarket, I've often heard parents hurling criticism or hostility at their little children. These verbal spears may be the result of fatigue or frustration, but they instantly deflate the child's spirits.

Almost all of us remember particularly stinging comments of a parent, teacher, friend, or family member. We may forget most of our day-to-day experiences, but we clearly remember being cut to the quick by words. For many of us, the hurt is sealed forever in our memories.

Yet if we think about it for a moment or two, we can probably recall uplifting comments from people we admired or loved that still make us smile and feel warm inside. For example, I remember the *one* compliment a coach gave me in front of the team as though it happened only moments ago. (Yes, I'm a "words of affirmation" kind of guy!)

So I'd like to ask two personal questions: Do you nurture your children through the power of affirming words? Or do you tend to be overly critical—using negative comments or harsh tones to put your children down?

Our children's nature is to believe what we tell them about themselves. If a father says to his son, "You are stupid," the boy is likely to believe it. If a mom tells her little girl, "You're ugly, and you'll never amount to anything," it's likely to happen. In contrast, think about the wonderful things that can happen when you positively affirm your children, when you verbally reinforce your love and appreciation.

I remember a wonderful little boy who was brought to me for evaluation for attention-deficit/hyperactivity disorder (ADHD) and failing grades. I immediately liked this creative, active second grader. I took a history, did an exam, and ran some simple tests. His mother brought him in for a follow-up exam to get the results.

I began, "All of the tests are normal except one."

His mom looked concerned. "What is it?"

"Well, the good news is, he's physically fine. He does not have ADHD, but he has a minor learning disability."

This little guy's mom stunned me with her response. "I knew it! He's stupid, isn't he?"

I could see the child's spirit break before my eyes. I suspected he had been told this many times before. It was time for an emergency intervention.

"Not at all. In fact, I think your son is brilliant."

The mom and her son look shocked!

I continued, "Children with learning disabilities often think they're stupid, or their parents or teachers tell them they're stupid. Now I want you both to listen to me very carefully."

I paused, leaned over, and looked directly into the little boy's eyes. "You are not stupid! You are brilliant! And you are *very* unique."

I paused for a moment and then looked at the mom. "Learning disabled does not mean stupid. It simply means that he has a different way of learning and processing information than his classmates. His trouble learning means we haven't yet discovered the learning style that works best for him."

I could see she was hearing what I was saying.

"Imagine having something really important to communicate but not being able to do it. Imagine not being able to focus your attention because you don't know how. Imagine trying to read or to do math but not being able to make sense of the letters or numbers. How would you feel?"

His mom bowed her head and whispered, "Stupid."

"He's not!" I emphasized. "He's gifted and creative and intelligent. We just need to help him figure out how he learns."

I could see the little guy's eyes light up. Finally someone understood him!

By the way, he recently graduated from college with honors and is entering graduate school. He credited his success to his biggest cheerleaders in life—his mom and dad.

No matter how much we parents want to use the power of words to nurture our children's confidence and concept of self, we will occasionally fail. All of us parents have made the costly mistake of wounding our children with critical or harsh words. Usually we knew we were wrong the moment the barbs left our tongues, but it was too late. Dr. James Dobson wrote about this type of mistake in his book *Bringing Up Boys:*

> If we tried for a hundred years, we couldn't take back a single remark. . . . The scary thing for us parents is that we never know when the mental videotape is running during our interactions with children and teens. A comment that means little to us at the time may "stick" and be repeated long after we are dead and gone. By contrast, the warm and affirming things we say about our sons may be a source of satisfaction for decades. Again, it is all in the power of words.

What should we do after we lose control and say something that deeply wounds our children? We need to seek to repair the damage and dress the wound as quickly as possible, before infection sets in. Talk to your child about what happened. Ask for forgiveness. The apostle Paul's advice of nearly two thousand years ago is still the best remedy: "Do not let the sun go down while you are still angry."

Allow Your Children to Make Their Own Healthy Choices

Our job as parents is to help our children realize their abilities and to instill a self-concept that enables them to develop their passion and pursue the destiny for which they were created. A key aspect of this process centers on allowing your children to choose what they think is best as opposed to choosing for them what you would prefer. It may mean allowing your children to pursue activities in which they are interested—even though they may not excel at them and may even fail. In the process, children become more familiar with their uniqueness, learn resilience when faced with challenges, and gain confidence to face new situations.

I'll never forget the day Kate announced that she wanted to take a shot at gymnastics because her best friends were dancers and gymnasts. Barb and I knew Kate was no gymnast. Because of cerebral palsy, her left side was spastic. She could walk, but running was difficult and awkward. Instead of berating or discouraging her, however, Barb and I talked to her about her disability and how it might make gymnastics more difficult. Kate, however, was *not* to be dissuaded.

I explained the situation to Ralph, a local gymnastics coach. He agreed it would be impossible for Kate to be a gymnast, but he concurred with our desire to let her try. "Dr. Larimore," he said, "why don't you pay for two lessons? I'll work with her on the tumbling mat. We'll see what happens."

During the first lesson, Ralph worked carefully with Kate to teach her a forward roll. It was very difficult for her. Ralph coached, he spotted, he encouraged. And, bless her heart, Kate really tried. Scott and I sat on the sidelines and rooted for her.

At the end of practice, Kate came running over to us. She was so proud of what she had learned. As we congratulated her on her accomplishment, Coach Ralph came over to commend her.

"Coach," said Kate, "thanks for teaching me and helping me. But I'm just not cut out for gymnastics, am I?"

He smiled and shook his head. "No, my dear, I don't think you are. But I'll tell you this. You're one brave and courageous girl. You keep looking. God has created you for something very special. It may *not* be gymnastics—but it *is* something."

Some parents would have viewed Kate's gymnastics lesson as a failure. To her, and to Barb and me, it was a success. By learning her limits, Kate was racking up more opportunities for achieving competence and feeling good about herself. And we were pleased to be able to recognize and affirm her efforts.

Dose of Wisdom

If your child has a long-term illness or disability, like our Kate does, the development of a balanced concept of self may be more challenging. Don't lose sight of the fact that there are more ways in which your child is like other children than different from them. Sure, you need to understand your child's uniqueness and limits, but avoid becoming so concerned for his or her safety that you deprive your child of enjoyable and beneficial experiences.

Building self-confidence in a child with a disability is not much different from doing so in a child without obvious disabilities. Provide as many opportunities as possible for success, and be ready to heap on extra helpings of encouragement and praise. Focus your comments on real accomplishments—on what the child can do, not on what he or she can't do.

Dr. Walt Larimore

Make Every Moment with Your Child Count

The day Kate, my oldest child, turned six years old, I spoke with my dad on the phone. "Walt, congratulations!" he said.

"For what?" I asked, a bit puzzled.

"Well, one-third of your life with Kate is over."

It took me a moment to realize what he was telling me: Kate would likely leave our home at age eighteen. Indeed, one-third of my up close and personal parenting time was gone. *That's it!* I thought. *I'm not about to let this time slip away.* Then and there I determined to spend more time with my children while I still could. To this day I'm thankful for my dad's reminder of how important and precious my time with my children was.

It was then that Barb and I decided to begin an intensive training program as parents, which we wish we had started when our children were younger. We read books on parenting. We spent more time with men and women who had successfully parented their children. We began applying most of the essentials you've been studying in this book. We discovered that these age-old principles worked. We began to see Kate and Scott develop and bloom as highly healthy children and then as highly healthy adolescents. We saw our relationship with them mature and become stronger.

Of course the parenting road was rocky at times. We were tested and at times beleaguered. Parenting is one tough job. But in the end, our hard work to raise highly healthy children produced wonderful fruit. Kate has graduated from college and moved into society as a highly healthy and productive citizen. Scott is still in college. They each have developed a wonderful and healthy concept of who they are. Their relationship with God, their parents, and their friends and colleagues are solid and profitable. We believe the world around our children will be better because they are there. For that, Barb and I are exceedingly grateful.

My prayer for you is that the fruit of your efforts to nurture your children's self-concept will be sweet indeed. If your children are going to develop a positive self-concept, they need *you*. They need your unconditional love, encouragement, understanding, and leadership. Most important, they need to spend quality and quantity time with you every day.

If you're willing to listen, I'd like to suggest an assignment to help you in this endeavor. Keep a small notebook or pad of paper and pen by your bedside. Each night for two weeks, jot down the number of minutes you spent talking or listening to each child who lives at home. Include only eye-to-eye time, not time watching television or time just being in the house together.

At the end of two weeks, you may be stunned to find out how little time you give each child. If that's the case, then I encourage you to make the decision I made when Kate was six years old. Don't let the time with your children slip away. Every moment you devote to them is an investment that will return benefits for at least the next four generations of your family.

Chapter Eleven

Engage in Healthy Activities

Rebecca was one of Barb's best friends when we lived in Kissimmee, Florida. Her children were younger than ours, and my wife, Barb, became a mentor for her. One day, early in their relationship, Barb suggested to Rebecca that they take her children to a local park to play while the moms sat by and visited. Rebecca looked at Barb quizzically. "Barb, why would we want to take them to play? They play all the time."

"What's wrong with that?" asked Barb.

"Well," Rebecca wondered aloud, "doesn't all play and no work spoil the child"?

Barb laughed. "Well, actually the saying is, 'All work and no play makes Jack a dull boy.'" Rebecca laughed at herself as Barb continued, "Rebecca, play is critical for growing children. It helps them in every way. Healthy play is—well—healthy."

Barb then explained to Rebecca that play is just one of many activities children need in order to become highly healthy. As a mother, Barb had learned that all children benefit from age-appropriate physical activities, activities that provide mental stimulation, activities that involve interaction with family members and others, and spiritual activities. A balanced mix of appropriate activities can have a significant positive impact on all the wheels of health. However, harmful activities (or *excessive* involvement in appropriate activities) can have a decisively negative impact on the wheels of health.

PLAY: IT'S A LOT MORE THAN FUN!

I remember how helpful it was for Barb and me to learn that children learn through play. At one time, doctors thought the development of a child's brain was pretty much complete at birth. We now know that only a few of the human brain's one hundred billion neurons are connected at birth and that a child's activities significantly affect continued brain development.

As a child experiences life, makes positive attachments to a mom and dad, and is stimulated by play and reading, the connections between the neurons in the brain form and strengthen. When reinforced by use, these connections become permanent. If these connections aren't used enough, they are damaged or eliminated. Repeated exposure to any stimulus in a child's environment, therefore, can have a positive or negative impact on his or her physical, mental, emotional, relational, and spiritual growth.

Medical research shows that there is a direct correlation between playful stimuli and early brain development in children. For example, functional brain scans of children show that when a story is read to a child again and again, a different part of the brain is stimulated each time. Other research has shown that playing peekaboo and playing with a mobile develop hand-eye coordination in the child. Researchers believe that the visual system continues its development during a child's early growth. So interactive play and age-appropriate activities are an important stimulus as children experience the world around them.

On the other hand, some activities deprive the brain of the experiences it needs to grow and develop. These include activities that encourage passivity (such as a child lying around for hours at a time without touch or stimulation) and maladaptive behavior (such as impulsivity or violence). Lack of interactive, stimulating activities deprives a child's brain of important opportunities to participate in social relationships, creative play, reflection, and complex problem solving—and this deprivation can lead to irrevocable negative consequences.

Sensory integration is the process by which a child's brain takes incoming information and organizes and interprets it so the child can respond to it appropriately. For example, through the tactile (or touch) sense, a child learns fine-motor movements such as pinching and grasping. A child's awareness of changes in head position and body movement help coordinate the movements of the eyes, head, and body. This sensory input is responsible for the muscle control that allows a child to manipulate objects, jump, run, and walk.

When children are not stimulated, touched, loved, and nurtured, there is a risk that sensory integration will not develop as it should. Lack of stimulation during early years of development (for example, a limited variety of foods and textures in the diet or limited opportunities for movement and exploration) plays a large part in contributing to sensory integration problems—which is why children who live in orphanages where they are left alone for long periods of time may display severe sensory integration difficulties.

Playing together as a family is one of the most highly healthy activities for children. It helps your children connect with you emotionally, relationally, and spiritually while developing physically and mentally. Play times with very young children include reading and singing to them and playing with them on the floor. With slightly older children, you can add activities such as playing in the yard, pushing them on the swing set, and throwing a ball.

As your children grow older, family fun activities will change. Elementary-school-age children enjoy walks in a park, visiting a zoo, and playing with puzzles and board or card games. You'll also want to make your home a fun, kid-friendly place where your children's friends will want to join in. This is especially important as children reach their teens. Time spent in family fun will provide abundant rewards for you and your children for years to come.

Dose of Wisdom

Dreams and beliefs are the fruits of sustained play. Play generates joy!

Edward Hallowell, M.D., child psychiatrist

I once asked a father of several highly healthy young men what he thought most contributed to the fact that they turned out so well.

"Walt," he replied thoughtfully, "we prayed for our boys and worked on their spiritual foundation. My career was never more important than my boys, and I was intentional about spending lots of time with them. My wife and I were always involved in their activities. We worked on finding ways to do fun things as a family. And as our boys grew, we made sure our home was a fun place for them to bring their friends. Our boys didn't need to leave home to find fun. They always knew it was right there for them at home."

Resource Box **Helpful Hints**

Just for Fun—

The Larimore Family's Five Favorite Activities When the Children Were Young

1. Playing a game or putting together a puzzle

2. Reading a good book together

3. Having a special family dinner where everyone helps

4. Going to the library together to pick out new books

5. Taking a walk together

A BALANCED DIET FOR THE MIND

Reading aloud to your child is one of the most important stimulations you can give your young child's brain. Repetitive reading stimulates the young brain in different areas. Each time you reread a story or a poem or sing another verse of the same song, your child's brain develops a bit more. So even if you've read *Jack and the Beanstalk* fifty times, keep on reading! Your child gets a little healthier every time!

Reading does more than stimulate brain development. It also helps promote language development. It helps young children learn to form words and to understand the relationship between words and objects. Reading with young children helps them learn to form sentences. Reading also teaches your children about the world in which they live. Through the world of books, the subjects of travel, fantasy, history, humor, adventure, and mystery can become a part of your child's life. And your child can enjoy it all in the comfort and security of sitting next to you or on your lap, which is a boost to self-esteem!

The benefits of reading truly are amazing. Most parents don't know it, but a love of reading is a more important indicator of academic success than a child's economic class. In one study of children from more than thirty countries, children from deprived backgrounds who enjoyed reading books, newspapers, and comics performed better on tests than children from more affluent homes. Reading for pleasure can also compensate for social problems that could otherwise adversely affect a child's academic performance. According to this study, being more enthusiastic about reading and a frequent reader was more of an advantage, on its own, than having well-educated parents in good jobs. Here are several important findings from the study:

- Fifteen-year-olds from impoverished backgrounds who enjoyed reading scored higher in literacy tests than children of well-off professionals who had little interest in reading.
- Students who didn't read as much achieved scores well below the international average, regardless of their parents' occupational status.
- Students who had access to a larger number of books in their homes had a tendency to be more interested in reading a broader range of materials.
- Parents who discussed books, magazine articles, politics, and current affairs with their children helped boost their children's literacy skills.

If your children are to reap the benefits of reading, your involvement is essential. Children are positively influenced to read when they see parents, siblings, friends, and neighbors reading. I've seen this firsthand in my family. Barb and her sister love to read. Their love of reading originated with their mom, dad, and aunts, who had seen Barb's grandmother reading. It's no surprise, then, that reading is one of our daughter's favorite activities.

How do you make reading a priority? You set the example! Read for yourself, and read to your children.

Resource Box   Helpful Hints

Getting the Most Out of Your Reading Time with Your Children

Here are some ways you can encourage good reading skills in your children (adapted from Children's World's Learning Centers' "Tips on Reading with Your Child").

- *Read early.* The years from birth to age eight are the most important period of literacy development. Experts suggest that parents begin reading with their child during the first weeks and months of life. Reading aloud and using interactive language are most important.

- *Read often.* Reading stimulates brain development in important ways, yet 50 percent of infants and toddlers are rarely read to. Experts suggest reading twenty minutes every day.
- *Read over and over again.* Children learn something new every time: new vocabulary, a different character, new meaning from the plot. It often takes at least four readings for a child to master the subject matter. Reading the same book also increases fluency.
- *Showcase books at home.* Surround a child with books—in the bedroom, bathroom, family room, and kitchen—and you will familiarize children with the purpose of books and how to use them. You don't have to spend a lot of money. Buy used books or buy books at discount stores. Or, like the Larimores, make frequent field trips to the library.
- *Model reading.* Let your child catch you reading. Read the mail, newspapers, and recipes out loud so your child knows that reading is a useful skill.
- *Make reading a family value.* Put reading before television and watching sports activities. Instead of a night out at the movies, have a family night at home with a good storybook. Read a chapter a night before dinner. Visit the library as often as you visit the park.
- *Build a vocabulary.* Books are the best vocabulary builders. To add variety, make sure your child has both nonfiction and fiction choices.
- *Make reading fun.* A parent's job is to make reading so enjoyable that a child will want to read all life long. Make it a warm, shared experience that connects love and learning. Parents provide the cozy lap, the good book, and the focused attention.

CHOOSE THE RIGHT ACTIVITIES FOR YOUR FAMILY

As important as reading is to a child's development and health, there are many other highly healthy activities you can enjoy as a family. For example, when I was beginning my professional career in family medicine, I chose to practice medicine while teaching medical students and residents and while conducting practice-based research. The research provided many opportunities to speak at medical schools and residencies. I rarely accepted a speaking invitation away from home unless my family could travel with me. Those family travel times were wonderful and fun experiences for our family.

Family travel exposed our children to a variety of museums, cities, customs, climates, geographical areas, and foods. Because our finances were limited, our children learned to budget and save, to shop and compare. These activities stimulated our children's intellectual, emotional, and relational development.

One of the things I always admired about Barb was how effectively she would balance activities. One week she'd take Kate and Scott to the library. The next weekend we might take a field trip to a museum or go on a hike as a family. One time the children would make a collage together, the next time we'd play a family kickball game. Barb not only varied the activities, she looked for fun, age-appropriate activities.

There are many healthy activities your family can enjoy together. The goal is for your children to enjoy these activities, to learn positive life skills, and to grow physically, emotionally, relationally, and spiritually. Take a look at the activity ideas listed below. You may already be doing some of these, and you may find other ideas that your family would like to try in the coming weeks.

Ideas for Family Activities

The chart below has a number of suggestions for engaging your children in activities that can be highly healthy. In general, the more passive activities tend to be less stimulating (physically, mentally, or relationally), while the more active and creative activities involve your child's physical and mental interaction. The more creative or active the activity, the more highly healthy it tends to be. However, healthy children need a balance of both types of activities.

Since many daily activities, such as driving across town, tend to be passive, parents can try to make them active and stimulating. For example, while riding in the car, children can count how many cars of different colors they see, or they can find license plates on cars from different states. (Just the other day, Barb and I were in the car together. She said, "There's a license plate from Hawaii. We've never seen one from Hawaii!" We both laughed.) A trip to and from the zoo or the movies can be made more stimulating by making up fun contests for the children. For example, Barb would encourage active involvement by asking the children to see how many names they could remember from the movie.

FAMILY ACTIVITY CHART

Home-Based Activities	
Indoor	**Outdoor**
More Active • Hobbies—baking, candle making, model building, needlework, crafts, rubber stamping, robotics, puppets, cooking, pets, model trains • Collecting—coins, stamps, postcards, etc. • Music, drama, dance, or indoor athletic training • Art—drawing, painting, origami, mask making, ceramics • Board games, puzzles, card games, blocks, word games	• Hobbies—birding, fishing, hunting, gardening, rocketry, model airplane flying, kite flying • Collecting—rocks, fossils, bugs, flowers • Art—outdoor drawing and painting • Games—Frisbee, badminton, bicycling, basketball, running • Soap bubbles
More Passive • Television—watching sporting events or movies • Computer games	• Cloud watching • Stargazing • Relaxing in the hammock
Activities Away from Home	
Indoor	**Outdoor**
More Active • Skating rink (ice or roller) • Bowling • Swimming pool, gymnasium • Library	• Swimming pool • Miniature golfing, riding go-carts • Hiking or camping at a local, state, or national park

More Active	• Music, drama, dance, or indoor athletic training and performance	• Sports—competitive running, bicycling, softball, soccer, volleyball • Snow sports—snowmobiling, snowshoeing, skiing, snowboarding • Water sports—fishing, water skiing, sailing, canoeing
More Passive	• Museums—aquarium, art gallery, science and industry museum, history museum, local specialty museum • Movie theater • Drama, dance, or musical presentation • Ethnic restaurant	• Zoo • Theme park • Train or boat (ferry) ride • Watching sporting events • Parades, fireworks, local festivals, ethnic community events • Visiting historical sites/reenactments

Choose Activities with Physical Health Benefits

Family activities not only increase a child's emotional and social health, but they can be crucial in developing a healthy physical wheel. They can help build a foundation of lifelong physical health for your children. Medical studies demonstrate that children who are exposed to exercise early in life are more likely to continue exercising for life. Sadly, the opposite is true, too. Parents may think their children will begin to exercise when they are older, but by age twelve or thirteen, a child is either turned on or turned off to physical activity.

Thankfully, increasing numbers of parents are choosing to exercise *with* their young children. Some families join health clubs or community centers that offer family workout sessions. Other families visit activity centers that offer batting cages, indoor climbing walls, or skating rinks. Some families play organized sports together, take family walks, or run or ride bicycles together several days a week.

Resource Box   ***Helpful Hints***

Make Fitness a Family Activity

Consider these tips for fitting fitness into your family activities:

- Build exercise into your existing routines. Park a reasonable distance from the mall entrance. Take the stairs instead of the elevator. At a soccer game, walk up and down the field rather than simply sitting on the sidelines.
- Think of easy, fun activities. Teach each other a dance. Take a ball to throw around in the park, or adapt a game to your family's needs.
- Give "active" gifts. Lots of kids want video games and CDs, but consider gifts that will make them more active—running shorts or shoes, a bicycle, a Nerf or Koosh ball.
- Weather got you down? Check out the roller- and ice-skating rinks. Or go to a local gym, bowling alley, climbing wall, or dance class.
- Select proper equipment for young children. Look for strollers with big wheels and strong frames that can endure ambitious outings. (For jogging, special strollers are necessary.) Backpacks, bike buggies, and bike seats enable young children to go with you until they are able to go under their own steam.
- Design a physical activity around your child's homework. If the homework involves math, incorporate counting into the activity. If it's American history, take a walk around historic sites (such as battlefields) or hike historic trails. If it's biology, identify trees, birds, and animals as you're out walking.
- Try new activities. You may look foolish, but it's good for your children to see you try new things—and even flounder a bit.
- Revive games from your childhood. Remember Red Light, Green Light? Duck, Duck, Goose? Simon Says?

- Take a brisk walk before doing homework or making dinner. Chances are the evening will go smoother, and you and your children will have lighter moods.

Choose Activities That Promote Spiritual Health

Family activities can also be crucial in enhancing children's spiritual health. In chapter 8, I discussed the impact a good spiritual foundation can have on your child's health. Now I'll share ways to incorporate fun spiritual activities into your family's daily routine—activities that can teach children the difference between right and wrong. One of my favorite suggestions comes from a group—Heritage Builders at Focus on the Family—that has developed hundreds of suggestions for family night activities. These activities can build up children emotionally, morally, and spiritually. I've excerpted an example from their "Family Night Tool Chest."

Resource Box   **Helpful Hints**

Tips for Successful Spiritual Activities

- *Make it fun.* Your children will always cherish the times of laughter. This is not an adult Bible study. Let the kids run, jump, or sing.
- *Keep it simple.* When you get complicated, you've missed the point.
- *Don't dominate.* Ask questions, give assignments, and invite participation.
- *Go with the flow.* If a question takes you in a different direction, great!
- *Mix it up.* Keep the sense of excitement and anticipation through variety. Skip the lesson on occasion; go bowling or out for ice cream.
- *Do it often.* Repetition is the best teacher.
- *Make a memory.* Create family night jingles that help recall the main theme.

SAMPLE FAMILY NIGHT ACTIVITY

Eggs-Cuse Me!

Main Point: All of us make a mess by doing wrong things.

Bible verse to review beforehand: Romans 3:23

What you'll need: Raw eggs, a small bucket of water, and a Bible.

Establish the ground rules: Ask all family members to agree to some basic guidelines. For example, you may suggest that everyone promises to participate in all activities and discussions and to refrain from being unkind or cutting down someone else.

Open in prayer: Have a family member pray, asking God to help everyone in the family understand more about him through this activity. Then begin!

Activity: Take your family outside to your driveway or a sidewalk area. (You may want to choose an area near your hose!) Indicate an imaginary line on the ground and have everyone stand with his or her toes along this line. Give each person one egg. Set the bucket of water about five feet from where family members are standing. Then explain that each person will toss his or her egg into the bucket—the goal is not to break the egg. Be sure to mention that anyone who breaks an egg must clean up the mess. Begin the tossing. If anyone makes it into the bucket without breaking his or her egg, have that person retrieve the egg, move back another foot, and toss again. Continue until each person has broken his or her egg. Then pull out the hose and have everyone help clean up the mess.

Share: Gather together and discuss the following:

- Was it easy or hard for you to hit the target? Explain your answer.
- What happened when you missed the target? (The egg broke; it made a big mess.)
- Is there any way to put the egg and its contents back together again? Why not?
- Let's compare our game to real life. How do we miss the target with God? (Answers may include: not doing what we know is right; disobeying parents, teachers, or employers; any other form of "missing the mark" or doing wrong.)

- How do we make a mess of things when we do or say wrong things? (We get in trouble; we get punished; we hurt other people; feelings get hurt; and so on.)
- How is it like breaking an egg? (We can't change the actions we've done, just like we can't put an egg back together.)
- Is there anyone who doesn't do and say anything wrong?

Read the Bible and Discuss: Read Romans 3:23 to your children. Discuss with them how this verse teaches that every single person makes mistakes and does wrong things. The Bible calls this "sin." The Bible teaches that sin is missing the target by not doing what God wants us to do. When we miss the target, we can make a big mess.

Wrap-Up: Gather everyone in a circle and take turns answering the question: What is one thing you've learned about God today? Then tell the children you've got a life slogan you'd like to share—a little phrase or jingle to help us keep in mind what we've learned.

Today's Life Slogan: *"When we sin, we disobey. So repent and go the other way."* Have family members repeat the slogan two or three times to help them learn it. Then encourage them to practice saying it during the week so they can talk about it at your next family night session.

Close in Prayer: Allow time for each family member to share prayer concerns and answers to prayer. Close your time together with prayer for each concern. Thank God for listening to and caring about us. You may want to start a family prayer journal to keep track of prayer requests; the answers can be recorded as evidence of God's working.

HELPING YOUR CHILDREN CHOOSE THE RIGHT BALANCE OF APPROPRIATE ACTIVITIES

As our children grow, they participate in an increasing number of activities outside the home. This is a healthy thing for maturing children to do. These activities allow children to meet and interact with other children. Through these activities children can be taught manners, cooperation, and sharing. In short, they can learn socialization skills that benefit them for life.

Our children often want to participate in far more healthy activities than time allows. Participation in too many activities is clearly detrimental to their health. As our children were growing up, Barb and I helped them evaluate the activities in which they wanted to participate. Whenever Kate or Scott came home with an idea about doing another activity, we'd sit down as a family to discuss the idea. I hope the process we used to evaluate activities can help you maintain a healthy balance in your child's life.

We usually limited our children to one or two extracurricular activities—especially if it involved practice time, training schedules, or time-intensive projects. We wanted our children to learn discipline and commitment—two highly healthy qualities that can result from participation in extracurricular activities—but also wanted them to have time for school, friends, church, and family.

You can guide your children toward being more highly healthy by helping them consider time commitments, schedules, homework, and other issues before committing to any activity. This is most important at the beginning of the school year when it's very tempting for children to choose several activities to join.

Some of the criteria we considered before committing to an activity may be helpful for your family, too.

- Barb and I discussed whether the activity would help our children learn more about themselves and what they'd like to be in the future. We weren't interested in activity just for the sake of activity. Most of the time we had these discussions with Kate and Scott present. We wanted them to know our thinking and reasoning, as well as to see us interact and make decisions as a husband and wife.
- We viewed activities that would develop our children's skills and abilities more favorably than highly competitive activities.
- We evaluated an activity in terms of the cost in money, time, and effort.
- We compared the cost to the time, money, and energy we had available. In many cases, prior commitments precluded adding another activity.
- All things being equal, we would let Kate and Scott choose their respective activities. We avoided pushing them into activities they weren't interested in or activities that met only our interests or expectations. We believed it was important to allow them to choose activities based on *their* interests, talents, gifts, desires, and available time.
- Once Kate and Scott became involved in activities, we viewed our role as being supportive, but not pushy.
- Once the school year was underway, our job was to watch for warning signs of overcommitment or too much stress. These signs include loss of interest in the activity, falling grades, loss of interest in and failure

to do homework, physical symptoms (headaches, fatigue, stomach pains), antisocial behavior, or injuries.

I realize these criteria may differ from family to family. But it's essential for your children's and family's health that you carefully evaluate and choose the right balance of activities. Through the years I've seen many parents who didn't do so. They were going ninety miles an hour and allowed (or, worse yet, encouraged) their children to do the same. This almost always resulted in stressed-out parents and children.

In fact, those of us who care for children medically are seeing an epidemic of stressed-out children. Many children in my practice were feeling the pressure of too many responsibilities and too little time. Stress in children is compounded by overcommitment. To allow (or require) a child to go from school to soccer practice and then violin lessons, followed by a fast-food supper in the car before going to a school or church social, then to arrive home exhausted and still have homework and chores to do, is a recipe for disaster. Stressed-out children may suffer from upset stomachs, overeating problems, sleep disturbances, depression, and headaches—and these are just the short-term consequences.

Many parents of my young patients seemed surprised by the amount of homework their children brought home every afternoon. They didn't account for adequate homework time before they started adding activities such as sports practices, music lessons, clubs, cheerleading practices, dance lessons, band practices, tutoring, study groups, youth groups, and so on. Without question, participation in these activities can be a great experience for most children, but there is no way highly healthy children can be involved in more than one or two at a time.

Dose of Wisdom

We need to make sure we're not expecting too much of [our children] at too early an age. Evaluate the number of activities they're involved in. If you wonder whether you're overprogramming your kids, you probably are.

Bill McCartney, founder, Promise Keepers

When children get involved in too many activities, the law of diminishing returns comes into play. Instead of feeling excited about the opportunity to excel in a particular area, overscheduled children may simply feel over-whelmed—which is why parents must keep a close eye on their children to ensure that their schedules do not become overloaded. Parents should watch for the common signals that children are experiencing high levels of stress:

- grinding or clenching teeth while sleeping, napping, or resting
- frequent headaches or stomach problems
- poor appetite or other changes in eating habits
- fatigue, trouble sleeping, or nightmares
- compulsive behaviors such as biting nails or licking lips
- poor concentration

You may be thinking, *Okay, you've got my number. What can I do to de-stress my children?* First and foremost, it's easier to prevent stress than treat it. If the stress levels from overinvolvement in activities are soaring in your home, you may need to cut back to allow for times of rest and family companionship. You may also need an attitude adjustment.

Let me illustrate what I mean by an attitude change. There was once a family that drove into a state park after a long journey. They were assigned a camping site and pulled into their spot while it was still daylight. As soon as the dad set the emergency brake, the car doors flew open and two children ran to the tailgate. Tarps, tents, anchor stakes, and lawn chairs sailed onto the ground. Within minutes, their campsite reached full readiness.

Next to them was another family that had arrived earlier in the day. That father watched as the other children worked feverishly to complete their tasks. Quite impressed, he wandered over and approached the recently arrived dad. "I couldn't help but notice how incredibly industrious your children are," he said. "How did you instill that kind of work ethic in them?"

The humbled father admitted, "Well, sir, thanks for the compliment, but you see, we have a system. No one goes to the bathroom until camp is set up!"

Activities don't have to drive the family agenda. Just as it's okay to slow down and relax on a camping trip, it's okay—even healthy—to build in some downtime where the family can have fun together and parents can show their children how important and valuable they are.

Before this chapter concludes, I'd like to share the importance of two other activities that can be highly healthy for children—family traditions and fam-ily vacations. These two activities can communicate in a powerful way how valuable and important your children are to you. They can play a crucial role in family togetherness and childhood health.

Resource Box   Helpful Hints

Resources for Family Activities

Books

Bennett, Steve, and Ruth Bennett. *365 TV-Free Activities You Can Do With Your Child.* Avon, Mass.: Adams Media Corporation, 1996. Illustrates how to make the most of free time, with suggestions ranging from arts and crafts to toy making to math and number games.

Cohen, Lawrence J. *Playful Parenting.* New York: Ballantine Books, 2001. Discusses the importance of recreation as a great way for children to explore their world and to work through stressful situations.

Hilton, Bob. *Weekend Dad: 101 Wonderful Ideas for Creating Memorable Time with Your Children.* New York: Prima Publishing, 2002. Includes community service ideas and science projects for fun, positive parent-child activities.

Miller, Thomas Ross, Beth Steinhorn, and Bruce S. Glassman. *Taking Time Out: Recreation and Play.* Woodbridge, Conn.: Blackbirch Marketing, 1995. Explores the world of play, games, and leisure without regard to age or background.

Wall, Amy. *The Complete Idiot's Guide to Family Games.* New York: Alpha Books, 2001. Tells parents how to institute a family game night with cards and other nonelectronic diversions.

Website: activeparks.org/ (part of the Active Network). A one-stop resource for sports and recreation participants. An inventory of more than 200,000 local recreation facilities in the United States, which allows citizens to find recreation facilities and associated activities in their area.

A HEALTHY DOSE OF TRADITION

My youngest brother, Rick, is an expert in the technical aspects of video and film production. Recently he took our family's 8mm films and transferred them to video and DVD media. For the first time in more than thirty years, I watched the videos and was transported back in time.

The films of every Christmas during our childhood recorded some of our most cherished traditions—putting decorations on the tree as a family, hanging stockings, going to midnight mass on Christmas Eve. Then, on Christmas morning, Mom would wake up all four boys. We'd have to put on our robes and slippers. When we were ready, she'd line us up, from the youngest (Rick) to the oldest (me), and out we'd march—to our utter delight. We'd open the presents, the glee apparent in our eyes. As I watched these films, a flood of emotions and memories overwhelmed me. I realized how important this tradition and other family traditions were to me.

Virtually all of us have some family traditions. They may be as simple as making French toast every Saturday morning or as intricate as special birthday or holiday traditions. Many family traditions are passed down from generation to generation, creating a link to your family's past. Others spring up on their own and establish themselves into the fabric of our families.

Traditions can strengthen family relationships now and can pave the way for future generations. As a family carries on its own traditions and rituals, family members develop a sense of oneness and meaning. Sharing common experiences tends to bring families together and keep them together. Traditions and rituals are what many memories are made of, and they pass easily from generation to generation.

Does your family need help in starting some new traditions? Many magazines publish special seasonal editions that feature decoration ideas, recipes, and holiday activities for families to enjoy. You may want to look for a book that discusses family traditions and how to develop them. The key is to select activities *your* family will enjoy. Some of them may become annual traditions that find their way into your hearts and your family scrapbooks, where they will be remembered and enjoyed for years to come.

As you develop your family traditions, include an activity that requires your children to write down their feelings. Doing so will provide a permanent, evolving record of their penmanship, memories, and emotions. You may want to start a gratitude journal, which you could bring out at each family gathering. Or you could keep a holiday guest book in which family members record their love and appreciation for each other.

Believing that our children needed a sense of security and a sanctuary in our home, Barb and I worked to institute family activities and establish traditions. These gave Scott and Kate a sense of rootedness and helped them realize that family and family relationships are essential to good health. As our children matured, some of our traditions changed. Some of our longtime favorites included the following:

- having Thanksgiving and Christmas dinners as a family
- taking summer trips to the beach
- dining together for breakfast and supper as often as possible
- attending family movie nights at the old Arcade Theatre in downtown Kissimmee, then going out to discuss the movie together
- playing card games and puzzles during holidays
- eating *pain perdu* (a type of Louisiana French toast) breakfasts every Saturday morning

Our traditions didn't always have to involve the whole family. Kate and Barb enjoyed making family scrapbooks together; Scott and I would hop into the truck and get a milkshake. These activities meant a great deal to all of us.

Resource Box			*Helpful Hints*

Keeping Your Family Traditions Healthy

Although family traditions are generally highly healthy, they can become unhealthy if we don't follow some basic guidelines (adapted from "This Is the Way We Always Do It," by Letitia Suk):

- *Good traditions are simple.* Activities that focus on people and values are usually long-lived. No matter how enjoyable they may be, ideas that are too elaborate or expensive may shorten tempers or have a short life span.
- *Good traditions are mutual.* If your spouse's family spent lots of money on gifts, invariably your family specialized in stocking stuffers. If the in-laws opened gifts on Christmas Eve, your family did so on Christmas morning. It's important for couples to talk about which traditions from each family you'll keep and which ones you'll uniquely create for your family.
- *Good traditions involve children.* Children love to participate in something they've helped plan. They like to have a special part that is theirs to contribute each time.
- *Good traditions need to be enjoyed, not endured.* This isn't as simple as it sounds. Many of us have endured traditions that could have been healthier (such as getting up

> at 5:00 a.m. to open Christmas gifts or cramming too many activities into one day).
>
> - *Good traditions need to be flexible.* Sometimes circumstances will alter even the most enjoyed and carefully chosen traditions. Only a few traditions survive the life span of a family. Circumstances such as college, marriage, or death of a loved one can end traditions. Sometimes age pulls the plug as children outgrow certain activities. For instance, no one carves pumpkins at our house anymore. No matter how long they last, traditions make us richer for having celebrated them together.

MAKE FAMILY VACATIONS A HEALTHY MEMORY

Like family traditions, family vacations have the potential not only to be healthy but also to be harmful to your child. I practiced family medicine in Kissimmee, Florida, for more than sixteen years. During that time, I cared for countless families whose vacations were highly unhealthy. Vacations tended to become unhealthy when families

- spent money they didn't have;
- tried to do too many things in too little time—leading them to become stressed-out, which reduced their immunity to anger, distress, and disappointment (on the emotional and relational wheels) and to infections (on the physical wheel); and
- planned every second of their vacations so they never had a few moments to relax and enjoy each other's company—seemingly forgetting how easily children get tired and how quickly tired children get fussy and irritate their parents.

When these things happen, guess what? The hoped-for fun family vacation turns into a disaster.

In contrast, healthy family vacations are relaxing and promote family togetherness, not family strife. An ideal family vacation reduces stress—that great robber of family health—and allows children and parents to relax together. Quality family vacations actually require less planning and more spontaneity and are designed for parents *and* their children.

Here are a few tips Barb and I have learned to apply when planning our vacation time:

- We never took a vacation we couldn't afford. It's always less stressful to plan a shorter, less luxurious family vacation than to have the stress of being in debt for months or years. Camping is an excellent low-cost family vacation that children love. (If this isn't your idea of fun, visiting a state or national park can be relaxing and inexpensive. Many parks rent inexpensive campers, tents, or cabins that can be fun to stay in.)
- Pick a relaxing spot. For us this was Barb's family beach house on the Florida panhandle. For decades, we have enjoyed a few days with no television, no radio, and no phone.
- Before the vacation started, Barb, Kate, Scott, and I would spend time discussing activities we would and would not do on the trip. By including Kate and Scott in the planning, we emphasized that this was their vacation, too.
- Don't plan every second of a vacation. My tendency was to pack our time with activities, but Barb wisely refused to let me do this. Yes, transportation and hotels should usually be planned ahead. Visiting some venues or events requires advance planning, but we tried to make the rest of a family vacation laid-back, casual, and spontaneous.
- Last, but not least, give yourself plenty of time to get home and prepare for work or school without a stressful rush. If you plan to return home with no margin for a flight delay or car breakdown, you may end your vacation more stressed-out than when you began. Barb insisted that we leave at least one day at the end of our vacation for sleeping in, unpacking, resting, and enjoying our children at home before returning to work. This day at home usually turned out to be one of our best vacation days!

Paul Batura, who capably handled the many research duties for this book, tells the following story of his family vacations. He graciously allowed me to share it with you:

As the youngest of five children, it is very easy for me to recall many memorable family vacations. We always assumed that every family routinely packed the station wagon, loaded the cooler, and headed to the ocean or the mountains for two weeks of unscripted fun.

Of course, our assumptions were incorrect. Although many families routinely take peaceful vacations, just as many—if not more—

do not. The reasons are many, but a popular and practical excuse relates to the financial burden of two weeks on the road. Given that reality, I once asked my dad how, given his modest income and growing family, he could afford the yearly trips that were, for our family, as steady as the sunrise. His answer floored me.

"Well," he said, "I was fortunate enough to work for a generous company that gave all employees yearly stock options. They would grant the options at Christmas, and just before the summer I would exercise them. That profit became our yearly vacation money."

I didn't realize how significant this sacrifice was until I was speaking with a group of my dad's former coworkers at his retirement party. Many of them had strategically held on to their options and exercised them much later in life. Because they waited to exercise their options, they had condos on golf courses and memberships in country clubs, and they took regular vacations to faraway places. They reaped wonderful rewards for holding on to their investments.

My dad? He had none of these things. He retired in the same house we grew up in, settled in with his wife of forty-seven years, and lives on a modest but sufficient fixed income that by no means rivals that of his former coworkers.

Who made the wiser investment? I'll let you decide. But the five children in our family have priceless memories of summertime fun. We have shared enough laughs to last a lifetime. Each of us knows what it means to have a highly healthy and enjoyable childhood. Not one of us would discount the dividends of our dad's investment.

Chapter Twelve

Cultivate Growth and Maturity

I was very interested in science by sixth grade, so I entered a project in the science fair at Highlands Elementary School in Baton Rouge, Louisiana. My project examined how and when to train plants to grow into one of three different shapes. Using bean plants (because they grew quickly), I demonstrated several points:

- If I waited too long to train the plants, they were more difficult to bend and more likely to resist training or to break.
- If I started too early or tried to train them too quickly, the tender plants were more likely to snap.
- If I began slow, consistent training early and continued the training as the plants grew, virtually all of the plants grew in the shape in which I wanted them to grow.

I had forgotten about this science project (for which I won a blue ribbon) until I took a college course in child psychology while simultaneously taking an Old Testament course. A verse in the Old Testament book of Proverbs caught my attention: "Train a child in the way he should go, and when he is old he will not turn from it." The Bible teacher explained that this verse meant each child is to be trained according to his or her *bent*—according to his or her temperament and giftedness, according to the way he or she is created. At the same time, the psychology professor explained how children must be trained through consistent parenting—not being too pushy or too lenient—that takes into account the child's uniqueness. What I had learned as a youngster about train-ing plants turned out to be an important life lesson.

From conception to adulthood, healthy children are always changing. How we parents train them—how we stimulate and direct their growth, devel-opment, and maturity—greatly influences their lifelong health. There is much we can do to bend, shape, nurture, and guide our children's growth and matu-rity without snapping or breaking them.

CHILDREN NEED CHEERLEADERS, NOT CRITICS

In chapter 10, we explored your child's uniqueness and love languages and how essential it is to understand these internal aspects in order to nurture your child's self-concept. You also need to understand them in order to be your child's cheerleader—to interact with your child in a meaningful way that encourages and cultivates growth. The ways we go about cheering on our chil-dren powerfully influence their health. Author and speaker Sharon Jaynes shares a delightful story about parental cheerleading:

> My nephew Stu began running on his school cross-country team when he was in the eighth grade. Since we lived 200 miles from his home, I didn't get to watch him run at his meets. I was delighted when I heard he had qualified for the state meet that was being held in my hometown. However, I heard the main attraction at Stu's races was not the runners, but his enthusiastic mother.
>
> I don't know if you have ever been to a cross-country race, but it is not exactly a spectator sport. Runners line up on the starting mark. A man fires a gun for the race to begin. Then the participants disap-pear down a trail in the woods, only to reappear some sixteen min-utes later.
>
> Before the race, my family stood on the sidelines, watching legs stretch, backs bend, and arms swing in an effort to warm up. Seventy anxious young men clustered around the starting line in ready posi-tion. The shot was fired into the air, and the herd of boys began their 3.1-mile jaunt through the woods. As soon as Stu's foot left the start-ing position, his mother, Pat, picked up her thirty-six inch mega-phone and began to yell louder than any woman I have ever heard.
>
> "GO STU!" she cheered, not once but at ten-second intervals. When he was out of sight, she ran to another strategic spot along the winding

trail where the runners would eventually pass by. And even though the boys were nowhere in sight, Pat continued to cheer, "GO STU!"

"Pat, do you have to yell so loud?" my husband asked.

"Yep," she answered. "GO STU!"

Steve inched his way a few paces behind us and pretended like he had no idea who we were.

"GO STU!"

I'll admit, it was a little embarrassing. She had no shame.

At one point she yelled, "GO STU!" and a man from across the park yelled, "HE CAN'T HEEEAAARRR YOOOUUU!"

"Pat, Stu can't hear you when he's deep in the woods. Why don't you let up a bit?" I asked.

"I don't know if he can hear me or not, but if there's a chance that he can, I want him to hear my voice cheering him," she answered. So for sixteen minutes, this little dynamo continued to pump confidence and inspiration into her son's heart.

Later, I asked my nephew, "Stu, when you are running on that trail in the woods, can you hear your mother cheering for you?"

"Oh, yes," he answered. "I can hear her the whole way."

"And what does that do for you?" I asked.

"It makes me not want to quit," he replied. "When my legs and lungs ache, when I feel like I'm going to throw up, I hear my mom's voice cheering for me, and it makes me not want to stop."

Isn't this a great story? To me, it conveys a wonderful picture of one of our most important roles as parents—believing in our children, encouraging them, supporting them, and cheering them onward and upward.

Compare this story to what my friend and mentor Dave Simmons experienced as a child. During high school, Dave was one of the best linebackers in his state. Yet after every football game in which he played, during the trip home, Dave's dad dissected every play and severely critiqued every mistake Dave made. The unrelenting criticism broke Dave's spirit and slowly eroded his love and respect for his dad. Dave needed a cheerleader, not a critic.

The cheerleader picture perfectly illustrates the impact a mother and father can have on their children. Their support and cheering can be felt and heard, no matter where a child is in life. A parent's cheers, or lack thereof, will echo from a child's past—from even a long distance. They can pump courage, encouragement, and confidence into his or her heart and soul.

Wise parents are cheerleaders on the sidelines of their children's lives. They know that their encouraging words, offered at the right time and in the right dose, can make the difference between their child finishing well or collapsing along the way. In contrast, an unwise or cruel parent provides the opposite. A parent's mean, malicious, or merciless words will cut to a child's core and snap or break the child's spirit. A mean-spirited cheerleader can stunt a child's growth and damage his or her path to maturity.

Former First Lady Hillary Rodham Clinton, for example, tells about her father, who never affirmed her as a child. When she was in high school, she brought home a straight-A report card. She showed it to her dad, hoping for a word of commendation. Instead, he said, "Well, you must be attending an easy school." Decades later, the remark still burns in Mrs. Clinton's mind. His thoughtless response may have represented nothing more than a casual quip, but it created a wound that has endured to this day.

As parents, we must realize that our cheerleading has the power to change our children's entire direction in life. We can choose to give them the awesome gift of positive cheerleading, or we choose to keep it from them. We don't need to buy our children the most popular and expensive brands of clothing or shoes or give them expensive or exotic vacations. We don't even need to buy them the newest computers, games, or electronic gadgets. *None* of these are crucial to a child becoming highly healthy. But we give our children a precious gift when we choose to feed their growth and maturity with a nourishing diet of encouraging words.

While I was writing this chapter, I asked Kate and Scott if they could recall any times when our parental cheerleading was particularly encouraging. Kate wrote this note:

> With my cerebral palsy, I wasn't able to walk well and running was difficult for me. Yet I wanted to try to complete a 5-K road race in our small town one July 4th. I decided to enter the race and do my very best.
>
> I wasn't able to run the entire 5-K, but I walked and ran. When I was about halfway done, I was beginning to feel exhausted and wasn't sure I could continue. At that moment, I heard you and mom cheering for me. "Go, Kate, go!" you yelled.
>
> Then, my brother, Scott, was at my side, encouraging me. "Come on, Kate. I'll run with you. We'll finish together."
>
> With the cheers of my family, I was able to finish the race. Even though I finished dead last, I finished it.

Not bad for a girl who had been told by her doctors when she was little that she would never walk. Yet without my family's encouragement and cheers, I never could have finished.

The gift of positive cheerleading can provide the spark your children need to accomplish things they might not otherwise accomplish. It can also leave positive memories that last a lifetime. Scott wrote about just such a memory:

My favorite memory of my dad as a cheerleader occurred during my sophomore year in high school. I was playing goalkeeper for the varsity soccer team. I knew my dad had taken time off from work to attend my game, and that meant so much to me because I knew how badly his patients needed him. But I think he knew how much more I needed him.

Toward the end of the game, our team was ahead by only one goal. Time was running down, and the other team was desperate for a score. They were coming toward me. I was so scared that I was going to let my team down, that I'd let my dad down!

All of a sudden, one of their players broke toward me, skillfully dribbling the ball. My heart began to pound, and I got prepared for the moment of truth. There was no one between him and me.

When he was within a few yards of me, he shot the ball toward the goal at an incredible speed. I didn't have time to think, only to react. Before I knew it, I was horizontal to the ground, stretching toward the ball. Somehow I barely touched it and deflected it.

At that moment, the referee blew his whistle. The game was over. We had won! My teammates all came running over to pile on top of me. It was one of the highlights of my youth.

But what happened after the game was even better. My dad gave me a big hug. We got into his old truck to drive home. He asked me questions about the game and let me talk. Then he said something I'll never forget. "Scott, until the day I die I'll never forget seeing you, horizontal to the ground, blocking that ball and winning the game. That picture will be in my mind forever. I'm so proud of you!"

I think of his words often.

I'm so glad Barb and I had these opportunities to bend, shape, nurture, and guide our children in their growth.

Helpful Hints

Cheers Every Parent Should Know—and Use

- Good job!
- I'm so glad you're my son [my daughter].
- Way to go!
- Wow! You look terrific!
- You played that song beautifully!
- You are a great child!
- You'll make a wonderful wife [husband] some day!
- You're going to be a great mom [dad].
- Thanks for cleaning your room.
- Look at those muscles. You're so strong!
- I love being able to trust you.
- Being with you [talking with you] lights up my day.
- One of the favorite parts of my day is picking you up from school.
- I missed being with you this morning.
- I'm proud of you!
- I knew you could do it!
- God made an incredible masterpiece when he made you.
- You are a treasure!
- I'm always behind you.
- I think it's neat we can talk about anything.
- I'm praying for you.
- You're a joy.
- You're amazing! How did you get so smart?
- That was so creative!
- Hurray for you!
- When God gave you to me, he gave me a precious blessing.

QUIETING THE CHEERS YOUR CHILDREN DON'T NEED

In my experiences as a family physician (and as a parent), I think I've seen or heard nearly every possible negative cheerleading example. Three negative cheers seemed to be most common: *comparing siblings, demanding perfection,* and *making rash comments in anger.* Although these cheers can be devastating, we parents can learn to silence them before they ever leave our lips. When they do slip out, we can take positive steps to correct the damage and encourage our children to continue growing as they should. Let me show you what I mean.

Comparing Siblings

Sandy brought in her two children for their well-child visits. Megan, the more compliant child, was the oldest. Her visit was uneventful. Then I started to examine little Matthew, a strong-willed, hyperactive child. His exam was challenging, and Sandy came unglued somewhere along the way. "Why can't you behave like your sister?" she nearly screamed. Matthew immediately paused and began to cry. Sandy had broken his little spirit.

After the exam, I sent Matthew and Megan out to be with my nurse. I explained to Sandy the incredible harm that can come when we compare our children to each other, especially when we're angry. "Sandy," I said, "doing this almost always leads to bitterness and resentment. The effects of this criticism may last a lifetime. It breaks a child's spirit. It's almost never an effective tool for correction, behavior change, or teaching."

Sandy looked crestfallen. "I had no idea. What should I do now?"

Her desire to be a good parent encouraged me. "Rather than comparing Matthew with Megan," I recommended, "emphasize his uniqueness. Congratulate him for what he does right. Give him options. You could say, 'Matthew, you have so much energy. How about saving it until after the visit with Dr. Walt? Then we'll go spend some of that energy at the park.' How does that sound?"

Sandy smiled. She could see what I was saying.

I continued, "In addition, you could encourage Megan to help Matthew learn to cooperate."

During their next office visit, Sandy asked if the two children could be seen at the same time. What a difference six months made! Megan was Matthew's coach. Sandy just watched. It was unbelievable.

At the end of the visit, I turned to Matthew and complimented him. "Matthew," I began, "Dr. Walt is so proud of how grown-up you were today. I think you are one special little boy."

If only you could've seen his smile and watched his little chest puff out! Even more gratifying were the grins on Megan's and Sandy's faces.

Negative sibling comparisons can originate from people other than parents. No matter what the source, it's important to take corrective steps. For example, when Kate and Scott were at a summer camp, Tim, the youth pastor, overheard a counselor taunting Kate. This counselor had thought that comparing Kate (whose cerebral palsy made it difficult for her to do many of the physical activities at the camp) to her brother might motivate her. Instead, it deflated her. Kate began to envy her brother and resent God for allowing her to be "crippled."

After correcting the counselor in private, Tim met with Scott. They planned a way to work together to encourage Kate. After lunch they approached Kate and proposed that she climb a rock-climbing wall. Kate refused. She was certain she could never do it, and she knew she could never climb as well as her brother.

"I'll help you," Scott insisted. "I'll support on your left side (Kate's weak side), and I'll ask Jake to be by you on your right side."

"You *can* do it, Kate!" Tim encouraged.

So she tried.

The boys worked with her. Campers and counselors cheered her on from the ground. Her climb was slow and clumsy. Every time her hand or foot slipped, Scott gently guided it back into place. He coached, encouraged, and cheered. When she made it to the top, the entire camp went crazy. When Kate and Scott got back to the ground, they fell into each other's arms, weeping with joy. When we saw the video, Barb and I wept. Almost a decade later, I still can't tell this story without getting tears in my eyes.

An event that could have scarred Kate for life became an experience she—and we—will never forget. By having one sibling help create a solution for the other, the wise youth pastor nurtured the unique bent of each. Instead of causing injury, he brought joy.

Demanding Perfection

When it comes to training children, striving for perfection is a perfect recipe for disaster. Perfectionism is often mistakenly viewed as desirable, or even necessary, for success. Recent studies, however, show that perfectionism actually interferes with success and health. The desire to be perfect can rob children of a sense of personal satisfaction and cause them to fail to achieve as much as children who have more realistic strivings. Perfectionism has been linked to depression, eating disorders, and low self-esteem.

Perfectionism places children in a vicious cycle. Children with this trait learn that people value them because of what they accomplish. As a result, they learn to value themselves according to the approval of others—which leaves them vulnerable and excessively sensitive to the opinions and criticism of others.

In order to protect themselves from such criticism, these children may decide that being perfect is their only defense, and so they set unreachable goals. They fail to meet these goals simply because they were impossible to achieve. Failure was inevitable. The constant pressure to achieve perfection and the inevitable experiences of chronic failure reduce productivity, effectiveness, and joy.

This unhealthy cycle often leads perfectionists to be self-critical and self-blaming, which results in even lower self-esteem and an increased risk of anxiety and depression. At this point in the cycle, perfectionists may give up on their goals and set different, but also unreachable, goals. They think, *If I just try harder this time, I will succeed!* Then the entire cycle starts again.

This unhealthy cycle spills over to the relational wheel. Perfectionists tend to anticipate or fear disapproval and rejection in their relationships. Given such fear, they may react defensively to criticism, and thereby frustrate and alienate others. Without realizing it, they may apply their unrealistically high standards to others and become critical of and demanding toward them. So perfectionists often have difficulty being close to people and can experience less than satisfactory interpersonal relationships.

Whenever we set unrealistically high standards for our children, we set them up for the frustration and failure of perfectionism. It's surprisingly easy to do. Barb was much better at avoiding this pitfall than I was. I like things "just so," and children don't fit this type of mold very well, if at all.

One Saturday Barb asked five-year-old Scott to make his bed. Soon he ran into the kitchen, exclaiming, "Mom, come look. I've made my bed."

Barb was at the sink, so she asked me to go with Scott and see how he did.

When I walked into his bedroom, I was appalled! The bedspread was uneven, the sheets were showing, and the pillows weren't evenly spaced. It was a *terrible* job. How could I tell him? He seemed so proud.

"How'd I do, Dad?" he asked eagerly.

I was just about ready to let him have a piece of my perfectionistic mind! I was irritated that he had done such poor work and that I had to leave the work I was doing at the kitchen table. But just then I heard Barb's voice behind me.

"Oh, honey," she exclaimed, "I'm so proud of your effort!" Elbowing past me while sending me a dart of a glare, she continued, "Look at you. You're taking care of your room. I'm so proud of you!"

She continued, "Honey, do you think we could straighten the cover out a bit? Can I help you, or do you want to show me how you can do it?"

He looked at the bedspread, instantly saw what she meant, and exclaimed, as he jumped to fix it, "I can do it, Mom!"

And he did!

I was so embarrassed as I saw his little chest expand in pride and a cute smile spread across his face. He looked up at me. Sighing in the realization that I could have (probably *would* have) made a terrible blunder, I thought back to when I was his age. I smiled at myself as I said, "Scott, I could *not* have done better when I was your age."

It was a true statement.

It would have been a big mistake to force my perfectionism on my precious little son. It would have undermined his confidence. It could have broken his spirit and potentially left a scar for life. Thankfully, Barb taught me how to praise and thank my children whenever they pitched in. She taught me what was appropriate for them to be able to accomplish at each age. In this arena, she helped me become a much healthier parent.

I know from my own tendencies that we parents can learn to more gently guide our children toward accomplishing their best rather than demanding a level of perfection that may break their spirits. We can help our children learn to set reasonable goals that are based on their gifts, talents, and desires rather than on our expectations. We can help them set realistic, achievable goals that are just one step beyond what they've already accomplished. We can help them learn to take pleasure in the process of pursuing a goal instead of focusing only on the end result. We can help them enjoy the satisfaction of their accomplishments. All of these practices will help our children avoid the pitfalls of perfectionism and grow into highly healthy adults.

Resource Box   **Helpful Hints**

Warning Signs of Perfectionism

Perfectionist parents and children have similar warning signs. Here are a few:

- *Fear of failure.* For the perfectionist, failure symbolizes a lack of personal worth or value.
- *Fear of making mistakes.* Mistakes equal failure, but those who obsessively avoid mistakes often miss out on opportunities to learn and to improve.
- *Fear of disapproval.* Perfectionists fear they won't be accepted if they reveal their flaws. They believe perfectionism can protect them from criticism and rejection.
- *All-or-none thinking.* Perfectionists lack perspective. They can't see the value in a "B" when an "A" is better. Anything less than perfect indicates total failure.
- *Overemphasis on "shoulds."* Perfectionists follow rigid rules and overemphasize "shoulds," rarely listening to their own wants and desires.
- *Believing others achieve success easily.* Perfectionists who view themselves as being inadequate believe that others achieve success with little effort, few mistakes, little emotional stress, and a lot of self-confidence.

Making Rash Comments in Anger

It's quite common for parents to make hurtful comments in the heat of anger. In most cases, these statements are an overreaction brought about when a child pushes a parent to the limit. A parent may be exhausted, frustrated, or angry when these destructive outbursts occur, but the verbal spears can wound a child for life. Parents who want to improve in this area simply must learn that the circumstances precipitating such comments are totally irrelevant. The only thing that matters is how incredibly destructive such comments are to children. Let's consider two examples.

Suppose, in a moment of anger, you scream at your six-year-old daughter, "I can't stand you! I wish I had never had you. I wish I could give you to someone else!" Or suppose your child brings home a report card with several bad grades. In your frustration, you exclaim, "I can't believe how stupid you are! You'll never amount to anything!"

In virtually every case, a child will carry the wounds from these kinds of outbursts for life. He or she will carry them in the deepest caverns of his or her subconscious mind and may replay them many times in conscious memory.

Your child probably will forget what he or she did to cause your eruption—even if it was something very wrong. But I guarantee that your child will never forget the words "I don't want you!" or "You are stupid!"

None of us are perfect, so we'll all experience times when we lash out and regret it. If you've made some of the same parenting mistakes I've made, my words may be convicting to you. But please understand, my purpose is not to make you (or me) feel guilty or remorseful. Rather, I want you to learn that the type of cheerleading you choose to use with your child has a lifelong impact. I trust that you want to be the cheerleader of a highly healthy child.

I've developed what I call my "philosophy of apology." When I goof and become aware of it, I apologize. It's an especially important practice for us as parents. If we make a mistake, if the anger that invariably comes during parenting spews out in the wrong way, then don't hesitate to make it right.

After the anger has subsided, spend a moment with God and admit to him that you were wrong and ask for his forgiveness. The Bible promises he will give it: "If we confess our sins, he is faithful and just and will forgive us our sins and purify us from all unrighteousness." Then go back to your child or spouse, and do the same. Confess and ask for their forgiveness. If you find that anger is a problem for you, seek help from a pastor or a counselor. Anger kills, and it is a problem great parents will want to root out.

LEARNING TO CHEER THROUGH THE UPS AND DOWNS

As a family physician I took great joy in watching parents respond to their child's growth and development. New parents looked forward to every new measure of their baby's growth—the first smile, first words, and so on. These early steps of growth and development have little risk, and parents can't imagine not encouraging their child to accomplish such milestones. In fact, if a child didn't reach a milestone within the appropriate time, the parents (and grandparents) would show up at my office demanding an explanation!

But as children grow and change, the process of growth and maturity isn't always pretty. It's not easy for parents to deal with the changes and risks that accompany growth. There will be ups and downs, for parents as well as for their children. It takes more effort and skill to keep on cheering. So while parenting is the most important responsibility we will ever have, it is also one of the most difficult jobs on earth.

Unfortunately, we receive little or no training in parenting. Most of us muddle along on our own. We usually do what our parents did—or we do the exact opposite, depending on our opinion of the parenting we received. One thing is certain: We will make mistakes. Sometimes we will cheer well; other times we will not.

I strongly encourage all parents to seek training in parenting skills. Such training is not reserved for "bad" parents; it is worthwhile for *every* parent. It helps us gain knowledge and learn practical skills that have been shown to improve the health of children. As we gain more parenting insight, wisdom, and skills, we see how we can be better parents. Barb and I took several parenting classes. Each one taught us new skills and gave us new ideas to implement in our home. Just as the training we do with our children helps them become the best they can be, training in parenting helps each of us become our children's best cheerleader.

I can't possibly pass along in one book everything you need to know to be your child's best cheerleader. I can't begin to explain all the training techniques that will help children become highly healthy young adults who are prepared to go out into the world and become everything their Creator designed them to be. But before I bring this book to an end, there are two essential elements I must bring to your attention: the tasks of letting go and of allowing mistakes.

Be Sure to Prepare to Let Go

There's a time for everything, and part of raising highly healthy children is knowing when to hold tight and when to let go. From the day they are born until the day they leave our homes as young adults, we have about eighteen years to teach our children to unplug from us and plug into life. We can't possibly do this at the right time or in the right way unless we *prepare ourselves* to do so. Humorist Erma Bombeck described this difficult process in a way that has been helpful to Barb and me, as well as to many parents I counsel. She compared the tasks of training and letting go of our children to flying a kite on a windy day:

> Mom and Dad run down the road, pulling the cute little device at the end of a string. It bounces along the ground but shows no inclination of flying. Eventually, with much effort, they manage to lift it fifteen feet in the air, but great danger suddenly looms. The kite dives toward electrical lines and twirls near trees. It's a scary moment. Will

they get it safely on its way? Then, unexpectedly, a gust of wind catches the kite, sailing it upward. Mom and Dad feed out line as rapidly as they can.

The kite pulls the string, making it difficult to hold on. Inevitably the parents reach the end of their line. What should they do now? Wanting to go higher, the kite demands more freedom. Dad stands on his tiptoes and raises his hand to accommodate the tug. The string is now grasped tenuously between his index finger and thumb, held upward toward the sky. Then the moment of release comes. The string slips through his fingers, and the kite soars majestically into God's beautiful sky.

Like it or not, the day will come when the kite will break free. Someday every parent will stand on tiptoes and stretch toward the sky, clutching the end of the string. It's best to let go when the time is right!

Just as parenting occurs in stages, depending on the age and ability of each child, letting go happens in stages. I think most parents begin the process of letting go way too late. Barb and I consciously began this process at the birth of each child. As I cut their umbilical cords, we prayed for the wisdom and strength to raise our children with the express purpose of launching them into the world. Gradually we shifted responsibility for their individual behavior from us to them. The process of letting go began the moment they were born and continues to this day.

The process of letting go is unique to each parent and child, so there is no absolute formula for parents to follow. Some children want to go to swimming lessons by themselves, for example, while others won't stick a toe in the water unless their mothers are sitting at the side of the pool. The key is to nurture growth gently and consistently in a way that suits each child—to figure out how to train a child according to his or her bent.

During the toddler stage, children become mobile and gain the ability to distance themselves from parents. They walk a balance beam between demanding to do things for themselves one minute and demanding that a parent do it for them the next. Parents begin letting go by allowing (or requiring) their children to do what they can do for themselves. We let them try, allow them to fail, and show them how to do things over and over again.

During elementary school, children still look to their parents for answers and information. Parents are not only their window to the world but a protective filter from the world. At this stage, parents provide opportunities for children to explore and pursue special interests through classes and extracurricular activities. Parents usually share with teachers and others in the community the responsibility of educating their children. We let go by allowing our children to participate, while we stand by to watch and to support them.

During adolescence, children begin to practice their adult roles. These times can be like a roller coaster for parents and children alike. One day can be "high," when a teen has everything going for him or her. The next day, the teen may "bottom out" and desperately need your support, love, and advice. Parents must learn to stand by patiently (rather than impatiently), hopefully (rather than helplessly), and prayerfully (rather than despondently) as their teens struggle to define who they are, what they want to be, and with whom they want to spend their time. We begin to take on more of a coaching role by allowing our children to make choices within safe limits and to experience the consequences of those choices.

Then comes the day when the child, now a young adult, announces that he or she is leaving home. If the process of letting go has been a gradual one, both parent and child are prepared to meet the resulting challenges. The responsibility for nurturing physical, emotional, relational, and spiritual health has been shifted from the parent to the highly healthy young adult. From this point forward, the parenting role changes. Our children still need parenting, but in a different way, under different rules. Our job as parents is not over, but our involvement is now activated by our children's invitation.

Learning how to slowly let go helped Barb and me survive the uncertainties and challenges of watching our children grow up. Gradually letting go strengthened our connections with and love for our children and enabled us to steer them from being highly healthy children to becoming highly healthy young adults. This has brought us unimaginably rich joy.

Be Sure to Allow Mistakes

The person who said "No one ever learned anything by being right all the time!" was absolutely right! Learning to deal with mistakes and overcome difficulties is essential. Growth and maturity require children to learn new skills, make mistakes, and take risks. A highly healthy young adult must know how to do household chores such as laundry, cleaning, shopping, and cooking. He or she must be prepared to handle financial obligations that include budgeting and managing rent, insurance, transportation expenses, utilities, phone bills, and so on. These tasks will be less overwhelming if the young adult has been taught how to do these things and has been allowed to make some mistakes along the way.

By allowing our children to make mistakes, we allow them to learn. But in my practice, I constantly saw parents who simply didn't want their children to ever have to go to the School of Hard Knocks. I know it isn't easy to make mistakes or to watch mistakes being made. The School of Hard Knocks is, indeed, hard, but it is necessary. So I encourage you to allow some mistakes along the way.

Consider my son, Scott, for example. He has become a great cook. His recipes are inventive and the food he prepares is delicious. But his culinary skills resulted from many mistakes in the kitchen: a microwave on fire (reheating popcorn in a plastic bag with a metal twisty); very salty chocolate chip cookies (used salt instead of sugar); adding cinnamon to lasagna just to "see what it would taste like" (it was awful). As he experimented, he occasionally hit a home run. Best of all, we saw his creativity and vivid imagination expand with each "mistake."

Children must be allowed to learn from wise and not-so-wise decisions. Of course they need to avoid mistakes that result from laziness or carelessness. They must learn when it is important *not* to make a mistake. They should do all they can to prevent mistakes that could lead to danger or harm. So we must help them understand the difference between "good" mistakes and "bad" mistakes. Here are the criteria Barb and I used to determine which mistakes were "good" or "bad": A mistake was acceptable if it arose through experimentation and creativity, resulted from conditions beyond their control, or resulted from a lack of knowledge.

Growing, maturing children will make plenty of mistakes. When they do, we have to help them cope effectively. Consider these ways to help your children avoid perfectionistic tendencies and learn to have a more relaxed attitude about mistakes:

- Laugh at yourself when you make mistakes, but don't laugh at them when they make mistakes.
- Provide enough extra materials and supplies so your children can start over (and you can encourage them to do so) if they make a mistake.
- React calmly when mistakes happen. Take a deep breath and ponder this thought: *Is this a "good" mistake, an accident, or an act of willful disobedience?* If it's either of the first two, encourage your child with statements such as, "Hmm. That didn't turn out so well. Let's try again."

- Encourage your children to turn their mistakes into learning opportunities by helping them determine what they could do to avoid the mistake next time.

We greatly increase our children's chances for becoming highly healthy adults when we allow them to experiment and "spread their wings" under our supervision and training.

CHEERLEADING MAKES ALL THE DIFFERENCE

No matter where your children's journey takes them, they need to know you love them unconditionally. They need you to keep on cheering! This foundation of parental love and support enables them to step out and grow into the young men and women God created them to be. But your child needs informed, consistent, loving encouragement from you, not just empty praise. To provide this lifelong gift, you must know your child well. You must spend time with your child and learn what is important to him or her. In short, you must demonstrate to your child that you care by your words and actions.

My mom and dad surely showed me! My mom told me thousands of times how much she loved me and cared about me, but what I remember most is what she did for me. One of my most vivid memories of her love in action occurred in the basement swimming pool of the local YMCA.

My swimming skills were just emerging, and I was delighted to compete in the city championships. My mom, a nurse, told me she'd try to change her schedule in order to attend the meet, but she wasn't sure she'd be able to. As I warmed up, I searched the gathering crowd. My mom wasn't there. I remember my profound disappointment. I knew she had to work, but I wanted so much for her to be there. As the meet progressed, I still didn't see her, and my disappointment grew. Finally my event was called. As I mounted the starting blocks, I glanced at the crowd. There she was, smiling and cheering for me!

I'm sure I swam faster and more furiously than ever before, and I won the event. As soon as I touched the wall, I looked around. Mom's smile stretched across the room. Both arms were in the air as she danced up and down and cheered—for me! In her nursing uniform!!

I'll always remember her cheering that day. I remember her sacrifice in getting there. I remember the message that echoed in her actions: "I love you. You are important to me!" My eyes still get misty, forty-five years later, remembering that moment. She was there for me.

I don't think there is anything a parent can do that is more meaningful or positive for a growing, maturing child than to "be there" as that child's cheerleader. The odds that children will become highly healthy adults skyrocket when they have cheerleading parents who are there for them. Let me share an example from Michael W. Smith's book *This Is Your Time:*

> My closest friends started going to all the parties. I knew there was nothing for me there, but my friends wanted me to be a part of that scene simply because they were. Deep inside I knew that if I didn't join them at the parties, there was going to be a change in our friendship, and there was. . . .
>
> The main reason I was able to stand against the partying crowd was because I received the acceptance I needed at home. "Fitting in" still mattered, but I didn't crave it like some others did. I knew my parents loved me, and I respected the way they lived their lives. They stuck with me through the hard times and demonstrated a consistent, unconditional love so that I never strayed so far that I lost my way.

This is the type of highly healthy parenting that helps to ensure that our children don't lose their way. This is the type of parenting I hope this book has encouraged in you. I pray that the essentials discussed in this book will assist you in raising highly healthy children, who will become highly healthy adults, who will contribute mightily to the health of the world around them.

My career as a family physician has been rewarded with more than its fair share of blessings. I've published more than 350 articles in the technical and medical literature. I've taught medical students and residents across the country. I've lectured to physicians in many countries. I've been blessed to host radio and television shows and have been interviewed for hundreds of media stories. I've been honored to be listed in prestigious professional listings, and I've been given many awards. But none of these accomplishments rank with the privilege and honor of being Kate's and Scott's dad and their mom's husband, which has been the most important work in my life. Now, when folks say, "Oh, you're Scott's dad," or "Are you Kate Larimore's father?" well, I just couldn't be happier or more pleased.

I don't know about you, but when my life comes to an end, I can think of no accomplishment that will be more important than to have left behind two highly healthy young people. For Barb and me, to know that Kate and Scott are highly healthy—physically, emotionally, relationally, and spiritually—is our highest and most satisfying accomplishment. To see their spiritual health blossom is the most rewarding. The godliness our children demonstrate in their lives has "value for all things, holding promise for both the present life and the life to come."

My hope is that when your parenting days are done, you will share similar feelings and fruit. Highly healthy children almost always come from adults who want to be highly healthy parents. My prayer is that this book will assist you in reaching this goal.

APPENDIX 1: WHEN TO CALL THE DOCTOR

This excellent list was adapted from "When to Call the Doctor" by Donna D'Alessandro, M.D., and Lindsay Huth, B.A. (Not every physician will agree with this list, so be sure to review these recommendations with your child's physician or nurse. If symptoms are severe, or if they worsen or persist, call your doctor.)

VOMITING

If a child vomits once or twice without other signs of illness, you can probably treat your child at home. Go to my website (www.highlyhealthy.net) to read more about vomiting.

- Give clear liquids in small amounts. Slowly increase fluids as the child is able to keep them down.
- Add soft, bland foods slowly. Gradually work up to a normal diet.
- Call the doctor if vomiting increases or gets worse.
- Call if the child is vomiting and also has stomach pain.
- Call if your child is dehydrated (see "Dehydration" below).
- Call if vomit is green or if there is blood in the vomit.

DIARRHEA

Minor infections may cause a few loose stools. Most cases can be treated at home.

- Give lots of fluids.
- Call the doctor if your child has many loose stools.
- Call if there is blood in the stools.
- Call if a newborn has more than six to eight watery stools a day.
- Call if your child is dehydrated.

DEHYDRATION

Vomiting, diarrhea, and fever can lead to dehydration, especially in infants.

- Keep track of how much a sick child is drinking and urinating.
- A young child or infant should urinate at least every six hours.
- An older child should urinate at least three times every twenty-four hours.
- Call your doctor immediately if your child is dehydrated. Symptoms include dry mouth, dry lips, dry skin, no tears, dark-colored urine, weight loss, decreased energy, or a sunken soft spot on an infant's head.

FEVER

Many minor illnesses cause fevers. Most can be treated at home. Go to www.highlyhealthy.net to learn more about fevers, about how to take your child's temperature and treat a fever, and about when to call the doctor.

Without Medication

If your child is still eating, drinking, and playing, he or she may not need medication.

- Dress your child in lightweight clothing or take off his or her clothes in order to lose heat through the skin.
- Cover your child in a light blanket if he or she is cold or shivering.
- Keep your child quiet. Activity could make the fever worse.
- Give extra fluids (such as water, Popsicles, Jell-O, or juices). If the child doesn't want to drink, give whatever fluids he or she will agree to.

With Medication

Medication may help your child feel better but may not stop the fever.

- Give acetaminophen (such as Tylenol, Tempra, or Panedol) every four hours. Read the label and follow directions. Give your child the right amount for his or her weight and age.
- Check with your doctor before giving ibuprofen (such as Pediaprofen, Motrin, or Advil).
- Do not use aspirin for fever. It can cause serious illness, especially if your child has influenza or chicken pox.
- Your child may need a sponge bath if he or she has a fever over 104 degrees Fahrenheit (or 40 degrees Celsius) and it hasn't gone down

thirty to sixty minutes after getting medication. Use lukewarm water, not cold water. Never leave a child alone in the tub. Stop the bath if your child starts to shiver.

- Do not use rubbing alcohol on your child's skin. It can cool your child too fast or give him or her alcohol poisoning.
- Call the doctor if your child has a fever and also a stiff neck or a rash.
- Call if your child will not eat or drink or if your child has other symptoms that worry you.
- Call if an infant under three months old has a fever.

RASH

A rash can usually be treated at home if your child doesn't have a fever along with it. If your child has a fever and a rash, call the doctor. Smaller rashes, such as those confined to the diaper area, can usually be treated at home.

- If a rash covers a large area of the body, call the doctor.
- If a rash hurts, swells, oozes fluid, or appears infected, call the doctor.
- Call if the rash affects your child's genitals or face.
- Poison ivy can usually be treated at home. Ease itching with a cool, wet cloth. A doctor should see severe cases.

COLDS

Colds are viral infections that cannot be treated with antibiotics. They are usually minor.

- Treating your child's symptoms will help him feel more comfortable.
- Call the doctor if your child has an earache or difficulty breathing.
- Call if symptoms worsen after three to five days or last ten to fourteen days.

MINOR CUTS, SCRAPES, AND INJURIES

- Call the doctor if your child has a severe cut. A large cut, a deep cut, or a cut with edges that are spread apart may need stitches.
- Call immediately if your baby falls or is dropped from any height. If an older child has more than a bump after a fall, it's usually a good idea to call the doctor.

- Call if your child has any injury that makes movement of his arms, legs, fingers, or toes difficult.

MINOR BURNS

Most small, minor burns can be treated at home with first aid. A more serious burn needs medical attention.

- Hold the burned area under cool running water for ten minutes.
- If a burn blisters or opens any layer of the skin, call the doctor.

NOSEBLEEDS

Nosebleeds are common, especially in the winter. Most can be treated at home.

- Have the child sit up, tilt his or her head forward, and pinch the upper part of the nose. Hold for ten minutes without letting go. Repeat if bleeding hasn't stopped.
- Call the doctor if your child has many nosebleeds.

APPENDIX 2:
MORAL/ETHICAL ISSUES
RELATED TO VACCINES

Some people have questioned whether the use of fetal cells in the production of vaccines is moral and ethical. One of my foundational ethical principles is that human life is sacred from the moment of conception when a new, unique human being is formed. This is a position I will never compromise for the sake of "medical research" or for the good of "science."

Having said that, let me explain that a line of human cells (known as WI-38) used to grow viruses for research is believed to have begun from the tissue (cells) of a legally aborted fetus in Sweden. These cells are used in the production of the rubella portion of the MMR-II vaccine. Dr. Leonard Hayflick at the Wistar Institute (thus the WI in the name of the cell line) developed the WI-38 cell line in 1962.

A second cell line, MRC-5, has been used to develop the vaccines called Vaqta and Havrix (administered to prevent hepatitis A). The Varivax vaccine for the chicken pox virus has been produced from both the MRC-5 and WI-38 lines. As for the origins of MRC-5, the Physicians Resource Council of Focus on the Family has found that this particular cell line was developed from the cells of a preborn infant who was aborted by the mother for "psychiatric reasons," although specific details haven't been revealed. For references on the issue of tissue cultures being derived from an aborted fetus, see the note on page 321.

As tragic and potentially unjustifiable as these two abortions may have been, they were apparently not performed with the intent of carrying out scientific or medical research. Although I abhor the practice of abortion, using these cell lines to continue to develop vaccines does not necessarily constitute formal cooperation in the act of abortion. Killing an unborn child is an ethically distinct act from that of producing a vaccine after the abortion has already been performed. Furthermore, no ongoing abortions are required to continue production of these vaccines. Cell lines derived from fetal tissue can be duplicated and grown in culture for decades, and thus additional abortions aren't necessary to replenish the vaccine supply.

For these reasons, I join the vast majority of faith-based medical ethicists who don't believe that producing or administering a vaccine made in the past from the cells of an aborted fetus is an evil act. Beyond the shadow of a doubt, moral people should speak out against unethical and immoral practices. I would never justify conducting an immoral practice so that something positive can result. However, in this case I can recommend these vaccines to concerned parents who have an obligation to care for their children's health.

I think of this situation as being comparable to letting your child receive an organ from a murder victim. The crime that led to the organ's availability was awful, deplorable, and punishable. But the organ itself is useable, and its use does not, in my opinion, take on any immorality of the act that led to its availability. Nevertheless, I completely support individual conscience. Due to the complex and highly controversial nature of this issue, it's understandable that some parents will still feel uncomfortable utilizing vaccines that are the by-product of abortion.

To find more information on this topic, access my website at www.highlyhealthy.net.

APPENDIX 3: PEDIATRIC USE OF ALTERNATIVE HEALTH CARE

In this appendix I wish to amplify on my reasons for not recommending the inclusion of alternative health care providers on your child's health care team.

Let's look first at the issue of chiropractic care. Through the years, chiropractic care has separated into two camps: *traditional* chiropractors, who adhere strictly to the philosophy of locating and eliminating "subluxations"—misalignments of the spine (see page 101 for my conclusions about subluxations)—and *holistic* chiropractors, who combine musculoskeletal manipulation and adjustments with other therapies such as gentle stretching, trigger-point treatments, hot or cold treatments, nutrition counseling and therapies, supplement recommendations, and exercise programs. The majority of practicing chiropractors fall into the holistic category, which is split into two primary schools of thought: *isolationist* and *rationalist.* The isolationists believe they can prevent and treat most diseases without the assistance of other health care providers. Preferring to work in isolation, they have either a disdain for or an aversion to anyone in the traditional medical world. The science-based rationalists, on the other hand, wish to be part of a traditional health care team.

During my years of practice in Central Florida, some of my adolescent and adult patients and I benefited from the services of a holistic, rationalist chiropractor. The patients who most benefited had acute musculoskeletal injuries, especially some forms of neck and back pain. However, I never used chiropractic services for young children, and I join most child care experts in the belief that chiropractors have virtually no place on a child's health care team.

I would caution you about isolationist chiropractors who often recruit children (even infants) and families into receiving expensive, unnecessary, and potentially dangerous care. Although some chiropractors believe that "chiropractic adjustment is sufficient in the treatment of most ailments," and "there is overwhelming evidence that spinal adjustments should begin at birth and continue for life," I'm not aware of any respected medical studies that support these beliefs.

Parents must be aware that some practice-building programs for chiropractors are based on pediatric care. A chiropractic research foundation called the Traumatic Birth Research Foundation, for example, encourages women "to participate in a 'chiropractic mothers and mothers-to-be program' to spread the word about the benefits of chiropractic manipulation for newborn babies. The message conveyed is that failure to correct spinal subluxations at birth could result in disease later in life."

This is utter hogwash. No reputable scientific research supports these delusions. Yet some isolationist chiropractors even provide manipulation for an unborn child in the mother's womb, which could result in the placenta becoming separated from the womb and a baby dying in the womb.

Another problem with chiropractic care for children is that many chiropractors hold unscientific views about immunizations, even though the official policy of the American Chiropractic Association states that "the use of vaccines is not without risk"—and therefore it supports the conscience clause in compulsory vaccination laws—and the Canadian Chiropractic Association "accepts vaccination as a cost-effective and clinically efficient public health preventive procedure for certain viral and microbial diseases, as demonstrated by the scientific community."

While these statements are in line with prevailing medical opinion, they don't represent the views of significant numbers of practicing chiropractors in the United States. One small survey of attitudes toward vaccination among American chiropractors found that one-third of the respondents believed there was no scientific proof that immunization prevents disease, that immunization has not substantially changed the incidence of any major infectious disease, and that immunizations cause more disease than they prevent. A larger study found that only 30 percent of chiropractors in the Boston area promote immunization (the effectiveness of which is supported by high-quality studies), while 70 percent recommend herbs and dietary supplements supported by little or no research.

Because of the concerns discussed here, I do not recommend including a chiropractor on your child's health care team.

The growing interest in alternative medicine among adults has led some parents to wonder if there may be some applications they should make to their children's health care. Should echinacea, a popular but scientifically unproven remedy for preventing colds, be given to a child with a runny nose? Is garlic oil a better eardrop than commercial products made specifically for children? What about acupuncture for children with cerebral palsy, or megavitamin, herbal, or supplement therapy for children with ADHD?

In a 2002 survey, researchers found that 2 percent of parents in the United States use alternative medicine with their children. The most common alternative providers were chiropractors (36 percent), clergy or spiritualists (24 percent), and massage therapists (14 percent). The most common types of therapies were spiritual healing (27 percent) and herbal remedies (17 percent). However, studies of parents of children who have chronic or recurring illnesses reveal that as many as 70 percent use alternative therapies in addition to conventional therapies.

Kathi J. Kemper, M.D., associate professor of pediatrics at the Center for Holistic Pediatric Education and Research at Harvard Medical School, is concerned about children who undergo surgery after taking herbal remedies. She has noted that some herbal remedies increase bleeding during surgery. Others have expressed concerns that some herbal remedies, while safe for an adult, could be overwhelming for a child, and some remedies could compromise the child's immune system or cause an adverse reaction. While we don't have a lot of information on dosage and effectiveness of herbal remedies in adults, we have even less with regard to children.

Parents who may want to treat their children with alternative therapies should keep in mind that many alternative medicine practitioners have little conventional medical training. In Massachusetts, for example, half of the homeopathic practitioners involved in one study had no medical training, and their training in homeopathy ranged from twenty years to only *three weeks.*

Despite an overwhelming lack of evidence to support using alternative therapies with children, many practitioners actively promote it. Rosemary Gladstar, an herbalist who has written many popular books, states, "Contrary to what you may have heard or read, my experience has been that almost any herb that is safe for an adult is safe for a child so long as the size and weight of the child are accounted for and the dosage is adjusted accordingly"—a conclusion she bases on her years of experience using herbal remedies and not on any controlled scientific studies. Thankfully, at least she acknowledges that herbs affect people differently and could cause serious adverse reactions.

The problem is, reliance on experience and intuition when using herbal medicine may indeed lead to physical harm. For example, while Gladstar claims that children can use "gentle herbs" like borage and licorice, as well as "stronger herbs" like comfrey and chaparral, "with no residual buildup or side effects," comfrey and chaparral are extremely toxic herbs that should *never* be taken orally by adults, much less by children.

Alternative therapies may also have a spiritual impact. Herbalists often claim the healing power of herbs comes as much from spirits that reside in nature as from chemicals in the plants. Taking children to an herbalist may expose them to spiritual teachings and activities that could be harmful. Just consider that when Rosemary Gladstar examines a child, she says she will "pray and let the spirit of the herbs guide me."

Some alternative procedures may be harmless to try. For example, many practitioners believe that acupressure and acupuncture are generally safe for children, although the issue of whether they provide effective relief is unresolved. The University of Arizona Medical Center has been experimenting with aspects of alternative medicine for children. Although nothing is conclusive at this time, some therapies are starting to show positive results. For example, relaxation therapies are proving to be helpful in relaxing the muscles of children who have cerebral palsy, which appears to reduce or delay the deterioration that invariably accompanies the condition.

The conclusion I shared on page 103 of this book bears repeating: If you choose to add alternative, complementary, or herbal therapies to your child's health care, or if you seek the services of an alternative practitioner for your child, be sure to do so under the direction and supervision of your health care coach—your child's primary care physician.

Resource Box   *Helpful Hints*

Parents who wish to find out more about particular herbs, vitamins, and supplements have free access to the world's largest and most trustworthy database on herbs, vitamins, and supplements (The Natural Medicines Comprehensive Database) through my website at www.highlyhealthy.net.

NOTES

Chapter One: What Is a Highly Healthy Child?

23: *"The four 'wheels'"*: Adapted from Walt Larimore, M.D., *Becoming a Highly Healthy Person* (Grand Rapids: Zondervan, 2003), 34.

23: *"grew in wisdom"*: Luke 2:52.

27: *"parents echo Jesus' perspective"*: See Matthew 6:33.

27: *"What good will it be"*: Matthew 16:26.

36: *"For married parents of adopted children"*: Note that it's not possible to earn a full spoke here. Later in this book I discuss the possibility that adopted children are at greater risk than biological children for not becoming highly healthy (see pages 183–84).

Chapter Two: The Parental Role in Nurturing a Highly Healthy Child

43: *"I always smile"*: See Judges 13:2–25.

44: *"After all, among"*: Reported in "Breakdown on Family Breakdown," *Washington Times,* March 25, 2001, B2.

44: *"As of the year 2000"*: Reported in Eric Schmitt, "For First Time, Nuclear Families Drop Below 25% of Households," *New York Times,* May 15, 2001, A1.

44: *"Given these disturbing trends"*: Reported in "Breakdown on Family Breakdown," B2.

45: *"Elder concluded that"*: Cited in Marilyn Elias, "Families Provide Antidote to Unhappiness," *USA Today,* December 9, 2002, 11D; see Glen H. Elder Jr., *Children of the Great Depression: Social Changes in Life Experience* (Chicago: University of Chicago Press, 1974), reissued as 25th anniversary edition (Boulder, Colo: Westview Press, 1999).

45: *"These findings were even"*: Cited in Elias, "Families Provide Antidote to Unhappiness.

45: *"A survey of"*: CASA, Luntz Research, and QEV Analytics, "Back to School 1999—National Survey of American Attitudes on Substance Abuse V: Teens and Their Parents" (New York: The National Center on Addiction and Substance Abuse at Columbia University, 1999), 6; can be viewed on the Web at www.casacolumbia.org/usr_doc/17635.pdf.

46: *"A recent large-scale":* See David Popenoe, "The Top Ten Myths of Divorce" (New Brunswick, N.J.: National Marriage Project, Rutgers University, 2002); can be viewed on the Web at www.rhfinc.org.au/docs/ten.pdf.

46: *"It is interesting to note":* See Linda J. Waite et al., "Does Divorce Make People Happy? Findings from a Study of Unhappy Marriages" (New York: Institute for American Values, July 11, 2002); can be viewed on the Web at www.americanvalues.org/html/r-unhappy.html. Using a large, national sample, researchers followed a group of marriages in which the partners rated their marriage as unhappy. When interviewed five years later, 86 percent of the formerly unhappy couples that stayed with the marriage indicated that they were significantly happier. Indeed, three-fifths of the formerly unhappily married couples rated their marriages as either "very happy" or "quite happy." In contrast, only one in five of the unhappily married couples that divorced were either "very happy" or "quite happy" five years later.

47–48: *"Even a quick reading":* This list can be viewed on the Web at www .novaroma.org/via_romana/virtues.html.

49: *"In yet another description":* Galatians 5:22–23.

49–50: *"The virtues that parents":* Reported in Steve Farkas, Jean Johnson, and Ann Duffett, *A Lot Easier Said Than Done: Parents Talk about Raising Children in Today's America* (New York: Public Agenda, 2002), 17; can be viewed on the Web at www.publicagenda.org/specials/parents/parents.htm.

50: *"2000 Harris poll":* Harris Interactive, "The State of the Nation," February 3, 2000; can be viewed on the Web at www.harrisinteractive.com/news/ allnewsbydate.asp?NewsID=52; Barna Research Group, "Most Americans Are Concerned About the Nation's Moral Condition," April 30, 2001; can be viewed on the Web at www.barna.org/cgi-bin/PagePressRelease.asp? PressReleaseID=89&Reference=B.

50: *"public schools should teach virtues":* Stanley M. Elam, Lowell C. Rose, and Alec M. Gallup, "The 25th Annual Phi Delta Kappa/Gallup Poll of the Public's Attitudes Toward Schools," *Phi Delta Kappan* 75 (October 1993); the poll has a margin of error of +/- 3 percent.

50–51: *"difficult virtue to teach":* Reported in Farkas, Johnson, and Duffett, *A Lot Easier Said Than Done,* 18–19.

52: *"Elizabeth Pantley":* See Elizabeth Pantley, *Perfect Parenting* (New York: McGraw-Hill, 1998), xxxix.

53: *"listed a family vacation":* Erin McClam, "What Makes for the Best Quality Time," *Athens Banner-Herald,* July 19, 2002; can be viewed on the Web at gameday.onlineathens.com/stories/071902/ent_20020719009.shtml.

54: *"This pressure has left":* Reported in "Parents Delay Paying Bills to Treat Children," *Western Mail,* November 23, 2002, 29.

54: *Richard Woolfson:* Cited in "Parents Delay Paying Bills to Treat Children," 29.

54–55: *Mary Ainsworth:* Cited in Robert Karen, "Becoming Attached," *The Atlantic* (February 1990), 35.

55: *"less likely to use drugs"*: Reported in "National Longitudinal Study of Adolescent Health: Success in School, Healthy Relationships Can Offset Risky Teen Behaviors," *NASP Communiqué* 30 (November 2001): 3:55.

55: *"Dr. James Dobson"*: James C. Dobson, Ph. D., *Complete Marriage and Family Home Reference Guide* (Wheaton, Ill.: Tyndale, 2000), 379.

55: *"Roxanne Spillett"*: Cited in McClam, "What Makes for the Best Quality Time."

56: *"ten commitments of great parents"*: Todd E. Linaman, Ph.D., "Ten Commitments of Great Parents," in *Family Life Matters* online (Tucson, Ariz.: Family Life Communications); these can be viewed on the Web at www.flc.org/hfl/parenting/ptg-flm03.htm.

Chapter Three: Be Proactive in Preventing Physical Disease

63: *"Research shows that many children"*: See Stella M. Yu et al., "Factors That Influence Receipt of Recommended Preventive Pediatric Health and Dental Care," *Pediatrics* 110 (December 2002), e73; can be viewed on the Web at pediatrics.aappublications.org/cgi/content/abstract/110/6/e73.

63: *"American Academy of Pediatrics"*: See *ACPM Headlines* (electronic newsletter for members of the American College of Preventive Medicine, January 3, 2003); can be viewed on the Web at www.acpm.org/10303.htm.

65: *"Yet research shows"*: Reported in H. Juhling McClung, Robert D. Murray, and Leo A. Heitlinger, "The Internet as a Source of Current Patient Information," *Pediatrics* 101 (June 1998), e2; can be viewed on the Web at pediatrics.aappublications.org/cgi/content/abstract/101/6/e2.

65: *"Researchers in 2002 searched"*: Reported in P. Davies, S. Chapman, and J. Leask, "Antivaccination Activists on the World Wide Web," *Archives of Disease in Childhood* 87 (2002), 22–25; can be viewed on the Web at adc.bmjjournals.com/cgi/content/abstract/archdischild%3B87/1/22.

66: *"unvaccinated children are"*: Reported in D. R. Feikin et al., "Individual and Community Risks of Measles and Pertussis Associated with Personal Exemptions to Immunization," *Journal of the American Medical Association* 284 (December 27, 2000): 3145–50; can be viewed on the Web at jama.ama-assn.org/cgi/content/abstract/284/24/3145.

66: *"a dramatic example"*: See "Measles Outbreak in Germany; Docs May Be at Fault," (New York: Reuters Health online, April 16, 2002); can be viewed on the Web at www.sabin.org/news_apr16_4.htm.

67: *"children over age two"*: C. B. Bridges et al., "Prevention and Control of Influenza: Recommendations of the Advisory Committee on Immunization Practices (ACIP)" *Morbidity and Mortality Weekly Report Recommendations and Reports,* April 25, 2003; can be viewed on the Web at www.cdc.gov/mmwr/preview/mmwrhtml/rr5208a1.htm.

67: *Offit and Bell:* Paul A. Offit, M.D., and Louis M. Bell, M.D., *Vaccines: What Every Parent Should Know,* 2nd ed. (New York: IDG Books, 1999).

69: *"Consider these facts":* Reported in "Vaccine Myths" (reprint of chapter 16 of Offit and Bell, *Vaccines: What Every Parent Should Know,* Immunization Action Coalition [2000]), 2; these can be viewed on the Web at www.immunize.org/catg.d/4038myth.pdf.

70: *"English journal Lancet":* A. J. Wakefield et al., "Ileal Lymphoid Nodular Hyperplasia, Non-specific Colitis, and Regressive Developmental Disorder in Children," *Lancet* 351 (February 1998): 637–41.

70: *"A subsequent study":* John Bignall, "UK Experts Convinced on Safety of MMR," *Lancet* 351 (March 1998): 966. See also Brent Taylor et al., "Measles, Mumps, and Rubella Vaccination and Bowel Problems or Developmental Regression in Children with Autism: Population Study," *British Medical Journal* 324 (2002): 393–96; can be viewed on the Web at bmj.bmjjournals.com/cgi/content/abstract/324/7334/393. Two studies have been conducted—each being very different in the quality and analysis of data. The second study (disproving an association between vaccine and autism) evaluated five hundred children; the first study evaluated only twelve. The second study included statistical methods adequate to determine whether MMR causes autism; the first study did not. The second study carefully evaluated the effect of MMR when first introduced into Britain on the incidence of autism; the first study did not. So, in short, the second study was much better than the first study and enabled one to conclude that MMR and autism were not linked.

71: *"a study revealed":* See "Thimerosal in Vaccines: A Joint Statement of the American Academy of Pediatrics and the Public Health Service," *Morbidity and Mortality Weekly Report* 48 (July 9, 1999): 563; can be viewed on the Web at www.cdc.gov/epo/mmwr/preview/mmwrhtml/mm4826a3.htm. See also "Mercury in Vaccines: What We Know"; can be viewed on the Web at www.immunizationinfo.org/features/index.cfm?ID=34.

72: *Offit and Bell:* Cited in "Vaccine Myths" (reprint of chapter 16 of Offit and Bell, *Vaccines: What Every Parent Should Know,* 5; can be viewed on the Web at www.immunize.org/catg.d/4038myth.pdf.

72: *"study recently reported":* D. Salmon et al., "Health Consequences of Religious and Philosophical Exemptions from Immunization Laws: Individual and Societal Risk of Measles," *Journal of the American Medical Association* 282 (July 7, 1999): 47–53; can be viewed on the Web at jama.ama-assn.org/cgi/content/abstract/282/1/47.

72: *"One researcher claimed":* J. B. Classen and D. C. Classen, "Clustering of Cases of Insulin Dependent Diabetes (IDDM) Occurring Three Years after Hemophilus Influenza B (HiB) Immunization Support Causal Relationship between Immunization and IDDM," *Autoimmunity* 35 (2002): 247–53.

74: *"poor oral health":* See "Oral Health in America: A Report of the Surgeon General"; can be viewed on the Web at www.nidr.nih.gov/sgr/execsumm.htm.

74: *"Very young children were"*: Reported in Stella M. Yu et al., "Factors That Influence Receipt of Recommended Preventive Pediatric Health and Dental Care," *Pediatrics* 110 (December 2002): e73; can be viewed on the Web at pediatrics.aappublications.org/cgi/content/full/110/6/e73.

74: *"American Academy of Pediatrics"*: In its policy statement on "Oral Health Risk Assessment Timing and Establishment of the Dental Home" (*Pediatrics* 111 [May 2003]: 1113–16), the American Academy of Pediatrics includes these two in its list of recommendations: "3. Every child should begin to receive oral health risk assessments by 6 months of age from a pediatrician or a qualified pediatric health care professional. 4. Pediatricians, family practitioners, and pediatric nurse practitioners and physician assistants should be trained to perform an oral health risk assessment on all children beginning by 6 months of age to identify known risk factors for early childhood dental caries"; can be viewed on the Web at www.aap.org/policy/s040137.html.

74: *"American Dental Association"*: See American Dental Association, "Fluoride and Fluoridation"; can be viewed on the Web at www.ada.org/public/topics/fluoride/fluoride_article01.asp.

78: *"For physical training"*: 1 Timothy 4:8.

78: *"Never before has one"*: The National Commission on the Role of the School and the Community in Improving Adolescent Health, National Association of State Boards of Education, American Medical Association, *Code Blue: Uniting for Healthier Youth* (Alexandria, Va.: National Association of State Boards of Education, 1990).

78: *"Dr. James Dobson"*: James C. Dobson, Ph.D., *Bringing Up Boys* (Wheaton, Ill.: Tyndale House, 2001), 54–55.

Chapter Four: Build Your Child's Health Care Team

81: *"Isadore Rosenfeld"*: Isadore Rosenfeld, M.D., "Power to the Patient," *Parade,* (February 24, 2002), 4.

89: *"Office of Technology Assessment"*: Congressional Office of Technology Assessment, "Nurse Practitioners, Physician Assistants, and Certified Nurse-Midwives: A Policy Analysis" (December 1986), 5; can be viewed on the Web at www.wws.princeton.edu/cgi-bin/byteserv.prl/~ota/disk2/1986/8615/861503.PDF.

95: *"J. W. Pennebaker"*: J. W. Pennebaker, *Opening Up: The Healing Power of Confiding in Others* (New York: Morrow, 1990), 118–19.

96: *"The Bible encourages"*: See 1 Timothy 2:2; Titus 2:2–8.

97: *"prayer affects a wide variety"*: Reported in Harold G. Koenig, Michael E. McCullough, and David B. Larson, *Handbook of Religion and Health* (New York: Oxford University Press, 2001), 104–6, 151–52, 199–200, 247–49, 313–14, 368–69.

97: *"the strongest factors"*: Reported in M. M. Paloma and B. F. Pendleton, "Religious Domain and General Well-Being," *Social Indicators Research* 22

(1990): 255–76; and "The Effects of Prayer and Prayer Experiences on Measures of General Well-Being," *Journal of Psychology and Theology* 19 (1991): 71–83.

97: *"National Mental Health Association":* National Mental Health Association, "Key Facts and Statistics"; can be viewed on the Web at www.nmha.org/children/green/facts.cfm.

101: *"no scientific evidence":* See Stephen Barrett, "Chiropractic's Elusive 'Subluxation'"; article can be viewed on the Web at www.quackwatch.com/01QuackeryRelatedTopics/chirosub.html.

102: *"chiropractors do not have":* Samuel Homola, "Is the Chiropractic Subluxation Theory a Threat to Public Health?" *Scientific Review of Alternative Medicine* 5 (Winter 2001); can be viewed on the Web at www.chirobase.org/01General/risk.html.

102: *"American Academy of Pediatrics":* Reported by Kathi J. Kemper, M.D., associate professor of pediatrics at Harvard Medical School, in *AMNews* (American Medical News [March 27, 2000]); can be viewed on the Web at www.ama-assn.org/sci-pubs/amnews/pick_00/hlsb0327.htm.

102: *"Another survey found":* Reported in Susan M. Yussman et al., "Complementary and Alternative Medicine Use in Children and Adolescents in the United States," 2002 Pediatric Academic Societies Abstract; can be viewed on the Web at www.aap.org/research/abstracts/02abstract22.htm.

Chapter Five: Ensure Proper Nutrition

106: *"national survey of parents":* Reported in Steve Farkas, Jean Johnson, and Ann Duffett, *A Lot Easier Said Than Done: Parents Talk about Raising Children in Today's America* (New York: Public Agenda, 2002), 20; can be viewed on the Web at www.publicagenda.org/specials/parents/parents.htm.

106: *"nine out of every ten":* Reported in Farkas, Johnson, and Duffett. *A Lot Easier Said Than Done,* 17.

106: *"survey of over three thousand infants":* Mathematica Policy Research, "Feeding Infants and Toddlers Study" (commissioned for the Gerber Products Company and presented at the October 2003 meeting of the American Dietetic Association); reported in T. A. Badger, "Babies' Eating Habits Poor, Study Says" *Philadelphia Inquirer* (October 26, 2003); can be viewed on the Web at www.philly.com/mld/inquirer/living/health/7107178.htm.

107: *"rate had increased":* Reported in Harry Pellman, "Obesity in the 21st Century," *Pediatrics for Parents* 20 (May 2003): 4.

107: *"Centers for Disease Control":* "ADA: One in Three Children Will Develop Diabetes," Diabetes In Control Dot Com newsletter; can be viewed on the Web at www.diabetesincontrol.com/issue160/item1.shtml. K. M. Venkat Narayan, M.D., presented the findings at the American Diabetes Association 63rd Annual Scientific Sessions.

108: *"University of California researchers":* Reported in J. B. Schwimmer, T. M. Burwinkle, and J. W. Varni, "Health-Related Quality of Life of Severely

Obese Children and Adolescents," *Journal of the American Medical Association* 289 (2003): 14:1813–19.

108: *"Obese children may have":* See www.shoppersdrugmart.ca/english/ health_wellness/health_information/health_conditions/m-s/obesity/get.html.

109: *"watch five or more hours":* Reported in S. L. Gortmaker et al., "Television Viewing as a Cause of Increasing Obesity among Children in the United States, 1986–1990," *Archives of Pediatrics and Adolescent Medicine* 150 (1996): 356–62.

109: *"promote unhealthy foods":* See "Television Ads Promoting Unhealthy Food for Children," AAP NEWSFEED, August 2, 2001.

109–10: *"fifty minutes of exercise":* Reported in M. D. Becque et al., "Coronary Risk Incidence of Obese Adolescents: Reduction by Exercise Plus Diet Intervention," *Pediatrics* 81 (1988): 5:605–12.

111: *"Eric Schlosser":* Reported in Eric Schlosser, *Fast Food Nation: The Dark Side of the All-American Meal* (New York: HarperCollins, 2002), 4.

111: *"teenagers who ate with their families":* Reported in B. S. Bowden and J. M. Zeisz, "Supper's On! Adolescent Adjustment and Frequency of Family Mealtimes" (paper presented to 105th Annual Meeting of the American Psychological Association); can be viewed on the Web at www.sciencedaily .com/releases/1997/08/970821001329.htm.

111: *"National Merit Scholars":* Reported in Mimi Knight, "The Family That Eats Together . . . ," *Christian Parenting Today* (January/February 2002); can be viewed on the Web at www.christianitytoday.com/cpt/2002/001/ 3.30.html.

114: *"fewer than 1 percent":* Reported in Julie Stafford, "Chew on This"; can be viewed on the Web at www.healthwell.com/delicious-online/D_backs/ Jan_99/healthbites.cfm?path=hw.

114: *"from a vending machine":* Reported in Elizabeth Becker and Marian Burros, "Eat Your Vegetables? Only at a Few Schools," *New York Times,* January 13, 2003, A1.

115: *"1998 survey":* Reported in Judy McBride, "Today's Kids Eating More," (Agricultural Research Service [August 11, 2000]); can be viewed on the Web at www.ars.usda.gov/is/pr/2000/000811.htm.

115–16: *"children who drink too much cola":* Reported in R. Hering-Hanit and N. Gadoth, "Caffeine-Induced Headache in Children and Adolescents," *Cephalalgia* 23 (June 2003): 332–35; can be viewed on the Web at www.w-h-a.org/wha2/Newsite/resultsnav.asp?color=C2D9F2&idContent News=574.

116: *"breast cancer prevention":* Reported in Joanne F. Dorgan et al., "Diet and Sex Hormones in Girls: Finding from a Randomized Controlled Clinical Trial," *Journal of the National Cancer Institute* 95 (January 15, 2003): 2:132–41; can be viewed on the Web at www.jncicancerspectrum.oupjournals.org/ cgi/content/abstract/jnci;95/2/132.

116: *"Harvard Medical School"*: See Walter C. Willett, M.D., *Eat, Drink, and Be Healthy: The Harvard Medical School Guide to Healthy Eating* (New York: Simon & Schuster, 2001).

118: *"nine servings a day"*: Reported in Scott Gottlieb, "Men Should Eat Nine Servings of Fruit and Vegetables a Day," *BMJ* 326 (May 10, 2003): 1003; can be viewed on the Web at bmj.com/cgi/content/full/326/7397/1003/a?etoc.

119: *"Katherine Tucker"*: Reported in Valerie Green, "Introducing the New Food Pyramid: Researchers Believe There Is a Better Way to Eat," *Tufts Nutrition* (October 1, 2001); can be viewed on the Web at nutrition.tufts.edu/news/matters/2001-10-01.html.

120: *"Walter Willett"*: See Willett, *Eat, Drink, and Be Healthy,* 17.

120: *"substance known as acrylamide"*: Reported in "New Tests Confirm Acrylamide in American Foods," *CSPI Newsroom* (June 25, 2002); can be viewed on the Web at www.cspinet.org/new/200206251.html.

120: *"American Academy of Pediatrics"*: Reported in L. M. Gartner et al., "Prevention of Rickets and Vitamin D Deficiency: New Guidelines for Vitamin D Intake," *Pediatrics* 111 (April 2003): 4:908–10; can be viewed on the Web at www.aap.org/policy/s010116.html.

120: *"oral vitamin K"*: For an excellent summary of this controversy, see Mike Gunderloy, "Vitamin K for Newborns"; can be viewed on the Web at www.larkfarm.com/AP/vitamink.htm.

121: *"nutrition in childhood health"*: Maria Boyle and Colleen Kavanagh, "The Importance of Nutrition for Health and Disease Prevention in Children Ages 0–6" (California Food Policy Advocates); can be viewed on the Web at www.cfpa.net/obesity/0-6paper.pdf.

122: *"understand its many benefits"*: See Rebecca D. Williams, "Breastfeeding Best Bet for Babies"; can be viewed on the Web at www.geocities.com/tebe7/breast1.html.

122–23: *"American Academy of Family Physicians"*: See: K. Sinusas and A. Gagliardi, "Initial Management of Breastfeeding," *American Family Physician* 64 (2001): 981–8; and American Academy of Pediatrics, "Breastfeeding and the Use of Human Milk," *Pediatrics* 100 (1997): 1035–39.

125: *"fruit juice consumption"*: American Academy of Pediatrics, "The Use and Misuse of Fruit Juice in Pediatrics," *Pediatrics* 107 (May 2001): 5:1210–13; can be viewed on the Web at www.aap.org/policy/re0047.html.

129: *"children serve themselves"*: Reported in Jennifer Orlet Fisher, Barbara J. Rolls, and Leann L. Birch, "Children's Bite Size and Intake of an Entrée Are Greater with Large Portions Than with Age-Appropriate or Self-Selected Portions," *American Journal of Clinical Nutrition* 77 (2003): 5:1164–70; can be viewed on the Web at www.ajcn.org/cgi/content/abstract/77/5/1164.

129: *"food allergies"*: For more on food allergies, see www.parentcenter.com/refcap/health/ills&inj/atoz/2106.html; caima.net/TheFoodAllergyNetwork.htm; and www.cbsnews.com/stories/2002/01/31/health/main327019.shtml.

Chapter Six: Provide Adequate Protection

131: *"hazards in our culture"*: Cited in Steve Farkas, Jean Johnson, and Ann Duffett, *A Lot Easier Said Than Done: Parents Talk about Raising Children in Today's America* (New York: Public Agenda, 2002), 9.

131: *"too many dangers"*: Cited in Farkas, Johnson, and Duffett, *A Lot Easier Said Than Done,* 9.

131: *"recent national survey"*: Reported in Farkas, Johnson, and Duffett. *A Lot Easier Said Than Done,* 12.

133: *"Jenny was one such parent"*: In this book, as in all my books, the names (and sometimes the gender and ages) of those mentioned are changed, and their stories are usually significantly changed, to protect them from recognition.

135–36: *"Michigan Psychological Association"*: See www.michpsych.org/index.cfm ?location=100&subsectionid=71.

136: *"shaping a healthy child"*: Adapted from James C. Dobson, Ph.D., *The Strong-Willed Child* (Wheaton, Ill.: Tyndale House, 1978); can be viewed on the Web at www.family.org/pplace/toddlers/a0000024.cfm.

137: *"Dr. Dobson warns"*: James C. Dobson, Ph.D., *Complete Marriage and Family Home Reference Guide* (Wheaton, Ill.: Tyndale House, 2000); see the article on the Web at www.family.org/docstudy/solid/a0014842.html.

139: *"experts who teach"*: Reported in American Academy of Pediatrics, "Guidance for Effective Discipline," *Pediatrics* 101 (1998): 4:723–28; can be viewed on the Web at www.aap.org/policy/re9740.html.

139: *"1996 scientific conference"*: Reported in S. Friedman and S. K. Schonberg, "Consensus Statements," *Pediatrics* 98 (1996): 4:853.

140: *"Dr. James Dobson"*: James C. Dobson, Ph.D., *Solid Answers* (Wheaton, Ill.: Tyndale House, 1997), 144.

140: *"Diana Baumrind"*: Reported in Diana Baumrind, "Does Causally Relevant Research Support a Blanket Injunction against Disciplinary Spanking by Parents?" (paper presented at the 109th Annual Convention of the American Psychological Association [August 24, 2001]; can be viewed on the Web at ihd.berkeley.edu/baumrindpaper.pdf; see also www.berkeley.edu/news/media/releases/2001/08/24_spank.html.

141: *"spanking should never"*: M. A. Straus, "Spanking and the Making of a Violent Society," *Pediatrics* 98 (1996): 4:837–42; M. A. Straus, D. B. Sugarman, and J. Giles-Sims, "Spanking by Parents and Subsequent Antisocial Behavior of Children," *Archives of Pediatrics and Adolescent Medicine* 151 (1997): 8:761–67.

142: *"Robert Brooks"*: Cited in Karen S. Peterson, "Experts Offer Tips to Ease Children's Anxiety," *USA Today,* October 8, 2002, A3.

142–43: *"Sam Goldstein"*: Adapted from Sam Goldstein, Kristy Hagar, and Robert Brooks, *Seven Steps to Help Your Child Worry Less: A Family Guide* (Plantation, Fla.: Specialty Press, 2003).

143: *"In a recent survey"*: Reported in Farkas, Johnson, and Duffett, *A Lot Easier Said Than Done,* 9.

144: *"parents of young children"*: Reported in Steve Farkas, Ann Duffett, and Jean Johnson, "Necessary Compromises: How Parents, Employers and Children's Advocates View Child Care Today," *Public Agenda Report* (2000), 19; can be viewed on the Web at www.publicagenda.org/specials/childcare/childcare.htm.

145–46: *"Bob Smithouser"*: Bob Smithouser, "What to Do When Bullying Hits Home," *Plugged In* magazine (October 2002), 3.

146: *"only experience worse"*: Reported in "Talking with Kids about Tough Issues: A National Survey of Parents and Kids" (March 6, 2001); can be viewed on the Web at www.kff.org/content/2001/3107/summary.pdf.

146: *"Dr. James Dobson"*: James C. Dobson, Ph.D., "Raising Boys: Expert Advice on Bullying," Focus on the Family daily broadcast, October 25, 2001.

146: *"American Medical Association"*: American Medical Association, "AMA Calls On Physicians to Help Reduce Bullying," (June 19, 2002); can be viewed on the Web at http://www.jaredstory.com/ama_bullying.html.

146: *"A 1998 study"*: B. Weinhold and J. Weinhold, "Conflict Resolution: The Partnership Way in Schools," *Counseling and Human Development* 30 (1998): 7:1–12.

146: *"most teenage suicides"*: Reported in Christine Morris, "Rejection Could Lead to Violence, Psychologists Say," *Miami Herald,* March 7, 2001, A7.

147: *"bullying among girls"*: See Rachel Simmons, *Odd Girl Out: The Hidden Culture of Aggression in Girls* (New York: Harvest Books, 2003), 3.

147: *"Dr. James Dobson"*: James C. Dobson, Ph.D., *Dr. Dobson Answers Your Questions* (Wheaton, Ill.: Tyndale House, 1982), 260.

147–48: *"Bob Smithouser"*: Adapted from Smithouser, "What to Do When Bullying Hits Home," 3.

149: *"televisions in their bedrooms"*: Reported in Farkas, Johnson, and Duffett. *A Lot Easier Said Than Done,* 13.

149: *"cable or satellite television"*: Reported in Federal Trade Commission, "Appendix B: Children as Consumers of Entertainment Media: Media Usage, Marketing Behavior and Influences, and Ratings Effects" (September 2000); can be viewed on the Web at http://www.ftc.gov/reports/violence/Appen%20B.pdf.

149: *"heavy sexual content"*: Reported in "How Much TV Is Too Much TV?"; can be viewed on the Web at www.christiananswers.net/q-eden/edn-f009.html.

149: *"Kate Moody"*: See Kate Moody, *Growing Up On Television* (New York: McGraw-Hill, 1984).

149–50: *"Media in the Home"*: Reported in Emory H. Woodard, "Media In the Home 2000" (Philadelphia: The Annenberg Public Policy Center of the University of Pennsylvania, June 2000), 19; can be viewed on the Web at http://www.appcpenn.org/05_media_developing_child/mediasurvey/survey7.pdf.

150: *American Academy of Pediatrics*: American Academy of Pediatrics, Committee on Public Education, "Children, Adolescents, and Television," *Pediatrics*

107 (February 2001): 2:423–26; can be viewed on the Web at www.aap.org/policy/re0043.html.

150: *"negative social messages"*: Reported in Farkas, Johnson, and Duffett, *A Lot Easier Said Than Done,* 15.

150: *"Barbara Brock"*: Barbara J. Brock, "TV Free Families: Are They Lola Granolas, Normal Joes or High and Holy Snots?"; can be viewed on the Web at www.tvturnoff.org/brock2.htm.

151: *"How to Get the Best"*: Dale Mason, Karen Mason, and Ken Wales, *How to Get the Best Out of TV: Before It Gets the Best of You* (Nashville: Broadman & Holman, 1996).

152: *"decreasing their television viewing"*: Reported in Thomas N. Robinson, "Reducing Children's Television Viewing to Prevent Obesity: A Randomized Controlled Trial," *Journal of the American Medical Association* 282 (October 27, 1999): 6:1561–67.

152–53: *"George Gerbner"*: Reported in American Psychological Association, "Violence on Television—What Do Children Learn? What Can Parents Do?" *APA Online;* can be viewed on the Web at www.apa.org/pubinfo/violence.html.

154: *"Dr. Daphne Miller's WebMD article"*: Article can be viewed on the Web at www.cnn.com/HEALTH/9908/20/kids.tv.effects/.

156: *"Nearly one in five"*: Cited in Parenting with Dignity, "Warning Signs: Chat Rooms"; can be viewed on the Web at www.warningsigns.info/chat_rooms_warning_signs.htm.

156: *"FBI has warned"*: Cited in Parenting with Dignity, "Warning Signs: Chat Rooms."

156: *"some simple rules"*: Cited in Parenting with Dignity, "Warning Signs: Chat Rooms."

157: *"trouble in cyberspace"*: Adapted from Parenting with Dignity, "Warning Signs: Chat Rooms."

158: *"worry about protecting"*: Reported in Farkas, Johnson, and Duffett, *A Lot Easier Said Than Done,* 9.

158: *"survey of seventh graders"*: Rodney Skager and Gregory Austin, "Report to Attorney General Bill Lockyer, 9th Biennial California Student Survey 2001-2002: Major Findings: Alcohol and Other Drug Use Grades 7, 9 and 11" (August 2002), 4; can be viewed on the Web at www.safestate.org/documents/9th_css.pdf.

Chapter Seven: Nurture Family Relationships

164: *"Shirley MacLaine"*: Cited in John Kronenberger, "Is the Family Obsolete?" *Look* (January 26, 1971), 35.

164: *"David Popenoe"*: David Popenoe, *Promises to Keep* (Lanham, Md.: Rowman and Littlefield, 1996), 248.

165: *"Barbara Dafoe Whitehead"*: Barbara Dafoe Whitehead, "Dan Quayle Was Right," *Atlantic Monthly* (April 1993), 64.

165: *"Parental divorce"*: Reported in Jane Mauldon, "The Effects of Marital Disruption on Children's Health," *Demography* 27 (1990): 431–46.

165: *"Child Study Center"*: Reported in L. Bisnaire, P. Firestone, and D. Rynard, "Factors Associated with Academic Achievement in Children Following Parental Separation," *American Journal of Orthopsychiatry* 60 (January 1990): 67–76.

166: *"suspended from school"*: Reported in Deborah A. Dawson, "Family Structure and Children's Health and Well-Being: Data from the 1988 National Health Interview Survey on Child Health," *Journal of Marriage and the Family* 53 (1991): 573–84.

166: *"without their natural fathers"*: Reported in Rebecca O'Neill, "Experiments in Living: The Fatherless Family" (London: Civitas: the Institute for the Study of Civil Society [September 2002]); can be viewed on the Web at www.civitas.org.uk/pubs/experiments.php.

166: *"Children from broken homes"*: Reported in O'Neill, "Experiments in Living: The Fatherless Family"; see Dawson, "Family Structure and Children's Health and Well-Being."

166: *"Babies born to single mothers"*: Reported in D. K. Li and J. R. Daling, "Maternal Smoking, Low Birth Weight, and Ethnicity in Relation to Sudden Infant Death Syndrome," *American Journal of Epidemiology* 134 (1991): 9:958–64.

166: *"emotional problems"*: Reported in Nicholas Zill and Charlotte A. Schoenborn, "Developmental, Learning, and Emotional Problems: Health of Our Nation's Children, United States, 1988," *Advance Data from Vital and Health Statistics of the National Center for Health Statistics,* vol. 190, publication #120 (November 1990).

166–67: *"Judith Wallerstein"*: Reported in Judith S. Wallerstein and Sandra Blakeslee, *Second Chances: Men, Women and Children a Decade After Divorce* (Boston: Ticknor and Fields, 1989), xvii.

167: *"thirty-three-year study"*: Reported in Bridget Maher, "Patching Up the American Family," *World and I* (January 1, 2003), 56; can be viewed on the Web at www.worldandi.com/specialreport/2003/January/Sa22832.htm.

167: *"Several studies show"*: See O'Neill, "Experiments in Living: The Fatherless Family."

167: *"worldwide survey"*: Reported in World Congress of Families II, "Special Report: Results of a Global Survey on Marriage and the Family"; can be viewed on the Web at www.worldcongress.org/WCF2/Survey/Famcong.pdf. See also Terry Mattingly, "Take the 'Family'—Please"; can be viewed on the Web at tmatt.gospelcom.net/column/1999/11/10.

168: *"Louise Silverstein"*: Louise B. Silverstein and Carl F. Auerbach, "Deconstructing the Essential Father," *American Psychologist* 54 (1999): 6:397–407; can be viewed on the Web at www.dadi.org/apa1.htm.

169: *"National Fatherhood Initiative"*: Reported in Wade F. Horn and Tom Sylvester, *Father Facts, 4th edition* (Gaithersburg, Md.: National Fatherhood

Initiative, 2002), 16; can be viewed on the Web at www.fatherhood.org/ fatherfacts.htm.

169: *"studies show father love"*: Reported in R. P. Rohner and R. A. Veneziano, "The Importance of Father Love: History and Contemporary Evidence," *Review of General Psychology* 5 (2001): 4:382–405.

170: *"father-absent homes"*: Reported in Horn and Sylvester, *Father Facts, 4th edition;* can be viewed on the Web at www.fatherhood.org/fatherfacts/topten.htm.

170: *"children with involved, loving fathers"*: Reported in Horn and Sylvester, *Father Facts, 4th edition.*

172: *"Brenda Hunter"*: See Brenda Hunter, *The Power of Mother Love: Strengthening the Bond Between You and Your Child* (Colorado Springs: WaterBrook, 1999).

172: *"Jay Belsky"*: Cited in Gwen J. Broude, "The Realities of Day Care," *The Public Interest* (Fall 1996), 96.

172: *"T. Berry Brazelton"*: T. Berry Brazelton and Stanley Greenspan, *The Irreducible Needs of Children: What Every Child Must Have to Grow, Learn, and Flourish* (Cambridge, Mass.: Perseus, 2000), 47; see the book review at www.familyandhome.org/books/brazelton2000.html.

173: *"current research on teens"*: CASA, Luntz Research, and QEV Analytics, "Back to School 1999—National Survey of American Attitudes on Substance Abuse V: Teens and Their Parents" (New York: The National Center on Addiction and Substance Abuse at Columbia University, 1999), 4–5; can be viewed on the Web at www.casacolumbia.org/usr_doc/17635.pdf.

173: *"American Academy of Pediatrics"*: You can view on the Web the AAP statement (www.aap.org/policy/020008.html) and responses from the Family Research Council (www.frc.org/?i=AR02B3) and Focus on the Family (www.family.org/welcome/press/a0019476.cfm   and   www.family.org/ welcome/press/a0020031.cfm).

173: *"American Sociological Review"*: Reported in Judith Stacey and Timothy J. Biblarz, "(How) Does the Sexual Orientation of Parents Matter?" *American Sociological Review* 66 (2001): 159–83.

174: *"Research on homosexuals"*: See Paul Van de Ven et al., "A Comparative Demographic and Sexual Profile of Older Homosexually Active Men," *Journal of Sex Research* 34 (1997): 354; M. Saghir and E. Robins, *Male and Female Homosexuality* (Baltimore, Md.: Williams and Wilkins, 1973), 225; C. M. Hutchinson et al., "Characteristics of Patients with Syphilis Attending Baltimore STD Clinics," *Archives of Internal Medicine* 151 (1991): 511–16; Joanne Hall, "Lesbians Recovering from Alcoholic Problems: An Ethnographic Study of Health Care Expectations," *Nursing Research* 43 (1994): 238–44; Karen Paige Erickson and Karen F. Trocki, "Sex, Alcohol and Sexually Transmitted Diseases: A National Survey," *Family Planning Perspectives* 26 (December 1994): 261; R. Herrell et al., "A Co-Twin Study in Adult Men," *Archives of General Psychiatry* 56 (1999): 867–74; D. Island and

P. Letellier, *Men Who Beat the Men Who Love Them: Battered Gay Men and Domestic Violence* (New York: Haworth, 1991), 14.

174: *"lesbian coparent relationships":* Reported in Stacey and Biblarz, "(How) Does the Sexual Orientation of Parents Matter?" 159–83.

174: *"No serious scientists":* See A. D. Byrd, S. E. Cox, and J. W. Robinson, "The Innate-Immutable Argument Finds No Basis in Science," *NARTH* [a peer-reviewed electronic article] (September 30, 2002); can be viewed on the Web at www.narth.com/docs/innate.html; "Is There a 'Gay Gene'?" *NARTH* (September 30, 2002); can be viewed on the Web at www.narth.com/docs/istheregene.html.

175: *"the Bible indicates":* See Numbers 14:18; see also Exodus 20:5; Exodus 34:7; Deuteronomy 5:9.

176: *"rate of child abuse":* Reported in Federal Interagency Forum on Child and Family Statistics, "America's Children: Key National Indicators of Well-Being" (1997); can be viewed on the Web at www.childstats.gov/ac2001/pdf/special97.pdf.

176: *"Crime":* Reported in Cynthia C. Harper and Sara S. McLanahan, "Father Absence and Youth Incarceration" (working paper, Princeton University, Center for Research on Child Well-Being, 1999); can be viewed on the Web at crcw.princeton.edu/workingpapers/WP99-03-Harper.pdf.

177: *"Drug and Alcohol Use":* Reported in John P. Hoffmann and Robert A. Johnson, "A National Portrait of Family Structure and Adolescent Drug Use," *Journal of Marriage and the Family* 60 (August 1998): 633–45.

177: *"Education":* Reported in Elizabeth C. Cooksey, "Consequences of Young Mothers' Marital Histories for Children's Cognitive Development," *Journal of Marriage and the Family* 59 (May 1997): 245–61.

177: *"Poverty":* Reported in United States Census Bureau, "Poverty: 1999" (May 2003), 7; can be viewed on the Web at http://www.census.gov/prod/2003pubs/c2kbr-19.pdf.

178: *"five times more violence":* Reported in Kersti Yllo and Murray A. Straus, "Interpersonal Violence Among Married and Cohabiting Couples," *Family Relations* 30 (1981): 339–47.

178: *"1996 study concluded":* Cited in Norval D. Glenn et al., "Why Marriage Matters: Twenty-One Conclusions from the Social Sciences," *American Experiment Quarterly* (Spring 2002): 43; can be viewed on the Web at www.amexp.org/aeqpdf/AEQv5/aeqv5n1/aeqv5n1.pdf.

179: *"Religion that God our Father":* James 1:27.

179: *"Gary Richmond":* Gary Richmond, *Successful Single Parenting: Bringing Out the Best in Your Kids,* expanded edition (Eugene, Ore.: Harvest House, 1998).

180: *"remarriage divorce rate":* Reported in Stepfamily Association of America, "Stepfamily Facts"; can be viewed on the Web at www.saafamilies.org/faqs/index.htm.

181: *"Ron Deal":* Cited in Carol Steffes, "Building a Successful Stepfamily" (Focus on the Family's Parents' Place); article can be viewed on the Web at www.family.org/pplace/schoolkid/a0025574.cfm.

183: *"living with adoptive parents":* Reported in M. J. Coiro, N. Zill, and B. Bloom, "Health of Our Nation's Children," *Vital and Health Statistics–Series 10: Data from the National Health Survey* (1994): 1–61.

183: *"New Zealand study":* Reported in David Fergusson and John Horwood, "Adoption and Adjustment in Adolescence," *Adoption & Fostering* 22 (1998): 24–30.

183: *"1985 study":* Reported in Marilyn R. Ternay, Bobbie Wilborn, and H. D. Day, "Perceived Child-Parent Relationships and Child Adjustment in Families with Both Adopted and Natural Children," *Journal of Genetic Psychology* 146 (June 1985): 2:261–72.

184: *"living with unmarried mothers":* Reported in Wade F. Horn and Tom Sylvester, *Father Facts, 4th edition* (Gaithersburg, Md.: National Fatherhood Initiative, 2002), 166–67.

184–86: *"Meanest Mother":* Bobbie Pingaro, "The Meanest Mother in the World" (written as a tribute to her mother in 1967). Used by permission.

Chapter Eight: Establish a Spiritual Foundation

188: *"an intense hostility":* Reported in Steve Rabey, "Videos of Hate: Columbine Killers Harbored Anti-Christian Prejudice," *Christianity Today* 44 (February 7, 2000), 21; can be viewed on the Web at www.christianitytoday.com/ct/2000/002/10.21.html.

188: *"James Garbarino":* See James Garbarino, *Lost Boys: Why Our Sons Turn Violent and How We Can Save Them* (New York: Free Press, 1999), 154.

188: *"Dr. Garbarino's research":* Garbarino, *Lost Boys,* 157.

189: *"Andrew Weaver":* Reported in Andrew Weaver et al., "An Analysis of Research on Religious and Spiritual Variables in Three Major Mental Health Nursing Journals, 1991–1995," *Issues in Mental Health Nursing* 19 (April 1998): 3:263–76. See also L. S. Wright, C. J. Frost, and S. J. Wisecarver, "Church Attendance, Meaningfulness of Religion, and Depressive Symptomatology among Adolescents," *Journal of Youth and Adolescence* 22 (1993): 5:559–68.

189: *"a sense of hope":* Reported in John C. Thomas, "Root Causes of Juvenile Violence, Part 2: Spiritual Emptiness," *Citizen Link* (June 1, 1999); can be viewed on the Web at www.family.org/cforum/research/papers/a0007791.html.

191: *"meeting on school grounds":* Reported in Jeremy Leaming, "Federal Judge Supports Policy That Differentiates between Student Clubs" (April 8, 1999); can be viewed on the Web at www.freedomforum.org/templates/document.asp?documentID=8638.

192: *"spiritual fruit":* Galatians 5:22–23. In academic publications I've called this *positive spirituality* because of the positive impact it has on people, their families and society. See W. L. Larimore, M. Parker, and M. Crowther, "Should

Clinicians Incorporate Positive Spirituality into Their Practices? What Does the Evidence Say?" *Annals of Behavioral Medicine* 24 (2002): 1:69–73. See also M. R. Crowther et al., "Rowe and Kahn's Model of Successful Aging Revisited: Positive Spirituality—the Forgotten Factor," *The Gerontologist* 42 (2002): 5:613–20.

194: *"foundation of true spirituality"*: Reported in Harold G. Koenig, Michael E. McCullough, and David B. Larson, *Handbook of Religion and Health* (New York: Oxford University Press, 2001), 78–94.

194: *"likely to testify to having"*: See Barna Updates, "People's Faith Flavor Influences How They See Themselves" (August 26, 2002); can be viewed on the Web at www.barna.org/cgi-bin/PagePressRelease.asp?PressReleaseID=119& Reference=E&Key=evangelicals. Despite public vilification, most evangelicals have a healthy self-image. Evangelicals are almost universally "happy" (99%) and were by far the segment that was most satisfied with their present life (91%). What's more, evangelicals are the least likely to say they are "lonely" (8%), "in serious debt" (9%), or "stressed out" (16%).

194–95: *"Cassie Bernall"*: See Matt Labash, "Do You Believe in God? Yes," *The Weekly Standard* 32 (May 10, 1999), 23.

195: *"to have less depression"*: Reported in A. W. Braam et al., "Religious Involvement and Depression in Older Dutch Citizens," *Social Psychiatry and Psychiatric Epidemiology* 32 (1997): 284–91. See also A. W. Braam et al., "Religion as a Cross-Cultural Determinant of Depression in Elderly Europeans: Results from the EURODEP Collaboration," *Psychological Medicine* 31 (2001): 803–14.

195: *"Spiritual beliefs and prayer"*: See M. M. Poloma and B. F. Pendleton, "The Effects of Prayer and Prayer Experiences on Measures of General Well-Being," *Journal of Psychology and Theology* 19 (1991): 71–83.

195: *"religious involvement is related to"*: Reported in Koenig, McCullough, and Larson, *Handbook of Religion and Health,* 78–94, 382–97.

196–97: *"But the basic reality"*: Romans 1:19–20 (The Message).

197: *"2002 national survey"*: Reported in Steve Farkas, Jean Johnson, and Ann Duffett, *A Lot Easier Said Than Done: Parents Talk about Raising Children in Today's America* (New York: Public Agenda, 2002), 39.

197: *"George Barna"*: Reported in Barna Updates, "Teens and Adults Have Little Chance of Accepting Christ as Their Savior" (November 15, 1999).

198: *"Phillip Johnson"*: Phillip R. Johnson, "Teaching Your Children Spiritual Truth" (1996), 1; article can be viewed on the Web at www.gty.org/~phil/articles/children.htm.

198: *"Johnson describes children"*: Johnson, "Teaching Your Children Spiritual Truth," 2.

199: *"Hear, O Israel"*: Deuteronomy 6:4–9.

200: *"James Dobson"*: James C. Dobson, Ph.D., *Complete Marriage and Family Home Reference Guide* (Wheaton, Ill.: Tyndale, 2000), 218.

203– 4: *"Lynne Thompson":* Lynne M. Thompson, "Five Minutes with the Bible"; can be viewed on the Web at www.focusonyourchild.com/faith/art1/A0000273.html.

204: *"William Sears":* William Sears, M.D., and Martha Sears, R.N., *The Successful Child: What Parents Can Do to Help Kids Turn Out Well* (New York: Little, Brown and Company, 2002), 201–7.

205: *"James Dobson":* Dr. James Dobson, Ph.D., *Bringing Up Boys: Practical Advice and Encouragement for Those Shaping the Next Generation of Men* (Wheaton, Ill.: Tyndale, 2001), 253.

205: *"Children who attend church":* Reported in Barna Updates, "Adults Who Attended Church as Children Show Lifelong Effects" (November 5, 2001); can be viewed on the Web at www.barna.org/cgi-bin/PagePressRelease.asp?PressReleaseID=101&Reference=D.

205: *"Robert Putnam":* Robert D. Putnam, *Bowling Alone: The Collapse and the Revival of American Community* (New York: Simon and Schuster, 2000), 66.

205: *"regular worshipers":* Noted in Putnam, *Bowling Alone,* 67.

206: *"physical training":* 1 Timothy 4:8.

Chapter Nine: Connect with the Larger Community

210–11: *"Everyone must submit":* Romans 13:1–2.

211: *"Obey your leaders":* Hebrews 13:17.

212: *"Good Home Habits":* Adapted from ARA Content, "Good Home Habits Taught Early On Have Long-Term Benefits"; can be viewed on the Web at www.pioneerthinking.com/homehabits.html.

214: *"National Association for the Education":* Adapted from National Association for the Education of Young Children, "Teaching Young Children to Resist Bias" (1997); can be viewed on the Web at npin.org/library/pre1998/n00123/n00123.html.

216: *"According to experts":* Gleaned from Youth Service America, "Facts and Figures on Youth and Volunteering"; can be viewed on the Web at www.ysa.org/nysd/statistics.html.

216: *"Sheryl Nefstead":* Cited in Marilyn Gardner, "Volunteering—A Family Affair," *Christian Science Monitor* (1995); can be viewed on the Web at www.volunteerinfo.org/famvol.htm.

216–17: *"Gallup survey":* Gallup International Institute, "Family Volunteering: A Report on a Survey" (Princeton: George H. Gallup Institute, June 1994); can be viewed on the Web at www.volunteerinfo.org/famvol.htm.

217: *"Youth who volunteer":* Gleaned from Youth Service America, "Facts and Figures on Youth and Volunteering."

217: *"55 percent of children who volunteer":* Reported in Jennifer Griffin-Wiesner, "Youth See Benefits of Serving Others," Youth Update newsletter (May 1995); can be viewed on the Web at www.search-institute.org/archives/ysboso.htm.

218: *"child who starts kindergarten":* Reported in G. W. Ladd, "Having Friends, Keeping Friends, Making Friends, and Being Liked by Peers in the Classroom: Predictors of Children's Early Adjustment?" *Child Development* 61 (1990): 1081.

218: *"children who experience rejection":* Reported in J. G. Parker and S. R. Asher, "Peer Relations and Later Personal Adjustment: Are Low-Accepted Children at Risk?" *Psychological Bulletin* 102 (1987): 357.

219: *"Dropping out of school:* Reported in Parker and Asher, "Peer Relations and Later Personal Adjustment: Are Low-Accepted Children at Risk?" 357.

221: *"Here are some tips":* Adapted from U.S. Department of Education, "Helping Your Child Through Early Adolescence" (2002); can be viewed on the Web at www.ed.gov/parents/academic/help/adolescence/part9.html.

222: *"research suggests":* Reported in Wise Men and Women Mentorship Program, "The Facts about the Mentoring Relationship: A Small Act with a Big Difference"; can be viewed on the Web at www.mentorship-wisemen.org/MentoringFacts.htm.

223: *"adapted from mentoring facts":* Adapted from Wise Men and Women Mentorship Program, "The Facts about the Mentoring Relationship: A Small Act with a Big Difference."

224: *"national study of mentoring":* Joseph Tierney, Jean Grossman, and Nancy Resch, "Making a Difference: An Impact Study of Big Brothers/Big Sisters of America" (Philadelphia: Public/Private Ventures, 1995); can be viewed on the Web at www.lion-cybercare.org/ementor-pkkd/results/results_1.htm.

224: *"young boys as sexual partners":* Researchers Karla Jay and Allen Young reported that 73 percent of the homosexual men they surveyed had engaged in sex with boys sixteen to nineteen years of age or younger (Karl Jay and Allen Young, *The Gay Report* [New York: Summit Books, 1979], 70). Most homosexual men are not pedophiles, but many pedophiles consider themselves to be homosexual. A study of 229 convicted child molesters found that 86 percent of offenders who molested boys described themselves as homosexual or bisexual (W. D. Erickson, "Behavior Patterns of Child Molesters," *Archives of Sexual Behavior* 17 [1988]: 83.

225: *"John Andrews":* John Andrews, "Hold Them Tight," *Andrews' America Journal: Notes on Our Times* (February 2003); can be viewed on the Web at.www.andrewsamerica.com/dynamics/resultaa.php?article_id=133.

Chapter Ten: Instill a Balanced Self-Concept

228: *"sent two bullets crashing":* Adapted from William Manchester, *The Death of a President* (New York: Harper and Row, 1967), 91–102.

230: *"the false self":* John Eldredge, *Wild at Heart: Discovering the Secret of a Man's Soul* (Nashville: Nelson, 2001), 107–13; for more on the basic questions, see pages 39–57 in Eldredge's book.

234: *"Paul Meier":* Adapted from Frank Minirth, Paul Meier, Richard Meier, and Don Hawkins, *The Healthy Christian Life* (Grand Rapids: Baker, 1988), 102–3.

234–35: *"early life experiences"*: See Carnegie Task Force on Meeting the Needs of Young Children, "Starting Points: Meeting the Needs of Young Children" (1994); can be viewed on the Web at www.carnegie.org/starting_points/. See also V. R. Fuchs and D. M. Reklis, "Adding Up the Evidence on Readiness to Learn," *Jobs and Capital* (Summer 1997): 26–29.

236: *"poem written by David"*: Psalm 139:1–7, 13–16.

240: *"Herbert Birch"*: See Herbert Birch, Stella Chess, and Alexander Thomas, *Your Child Is a Person* (New York: Viking Penguin, 1965).

243: *"Gary Chapman"*: Gary Chapman and Ross Campbell, *The Five Love Languages of Children* (Chicago: Northfield, 1997), 164.

247: *"James Dobson"*: James C. Dobson, Ph.D., *Bringing Up Boys* (Wheaton, Ill.: Tyndale, 2001), 221

247: *"the apostle Paul's advice"*: Ephesians 4:26.

Chapter Eleven: Engage in Healthy Activities

255: *"several important findings"*: Reported in Organization for Economic Co-operation and Development, "Reading for Change: Performance and Engagement across Countries: Results from PISA 2000"; can be viewed on the Web at www.pisa.oecd.org/change/download.htm.

255: *"are some ways"*: Children's World's Learning Centers, "Tips on Reading with Your Child"; can be viewed on the Web at www.childrensworld.com/readingtips.html.

261: *"Family Night Tool Chest"*: Adapted from Kurt Bruner and Jim Weidmann, "Family Night Tool Chest," in *Basic Christian Beliefs* (Colorado Springs: Victor Chariot, 1998); can be viewed on the Web at heritagebuilders.com/weeklyactivities/a0000465.cfm.

269: *"This Is the Way"*: Adapted from Letitia Suk, "This Is the Way We Always Do It," *Focus on the Family Magazine* (2002); can be viewed on the Web at www.family.org/fofmag/sh/a0022978.cfm.

Chapter Twelve: Cultivate Growth and Maturity

273: *"Train a child"*: Proverbs 22:6.

274–75: *"Sharon Jaynes"*: Sharon Jaynes, "Becoming Your Child's Chief Cheerleader"; can be viewed on the Web at www.family.org/pplace/youandteens/a0019553.cfm.

276: *"never affirmed her as a child"*: Story cited in James C. Dobson, Ph.D., *Bringing Up Boys* (Wheaton, Ill.: Tyndale House, 2001), 219.

284: *"If we confess"*: 1 John 1:9.

285: *"gain knowledge"*: Reported in Jane Barlow and Jacqueline Parsons, "Group-Based Parent-Training Programmes for Improving Emotional and Behavioural Adjustment in 0–3 Year Old Children" (Cochrane Review), *The Cochrane Library* 4 (2003); abstract can be viewed on the Web at www.update-software.com/abstracts/ab003680.htm.

285–86: *"Erma Bombeck":* Erma Bombeck, *Forever Erma: Best-Loved Writing from America's Favorite Humorist* (Kansas City, Mo.: Andrews McMeel, 1997), 44–45.

290: *"Michael W. Smith's book":* Michael W. Smith, *This Is Your Time: Make Every Moment Count* (Nashville: Nelson, 2000), 91.

291: *"value for all things":* 1 Timothy 4:8.

Appendix 1: When to Call the Doctor

293: *"When to Call the Doctor":* Adapted from Donna D'Alessandro, M.D., and Lindsay Huth, B.A., "Pediatrics Common Questions, Quick Answers: When to Call the Doctor"; can be viewed on the Web at www.vh.org/pediatric/patient/pediatrics/cqqa/callthedoctor.html.

Appendix 2: Moral/Ethical Issues Related to Vaccines

297: *"references on the issue":* Merck and Company, "Manufacturing Insert for MMR-II, Varivax, Vaqta, and Havrix"; can be viewed on the Web at www.cogforlife.org/packageinserts.htm; "Gamma Globulin Prophylaxis; Inactivated Rubella Virus; Production and Biologics Control of Live Attenuated Rubella Virus Vaccines," *American Journal of Diseases of Childhood* 118 (1969): 2:372–81; S. A. Plotkin, J. D. Farquhar, M. Katz, and F. Buser, "Attenuation of RA 27–3 Rubella Virus in WI–38 Human Diploid Cells," *American Journal of Diseases of Childhood* 118 (1969): 2:178–85; S. A. Plotkin, D. Cornfeld, and T. H. Ingalls, "Studies of Immunization with Living Rubella Virus. Trials in Children with a Strain Cultured from an Aborted Fetus," *American Journal of Diseases of Childhood* 110 (1965): 4:381–89.

Appendix 3: Pediatric Use of Alternative Health Care

299: *"chiropractic adjustment is sufficient":* Cited in Samuel Homola, "Is the Chiropractic Subluxation Theory a Threat to Public Health?" *Scientific Review of Alternative Medicine* 5 (Winter 2001); can be viewed on the Web at www.chirobase.org/01General/risk.html.

300: *"Traumatic Birth Research Foundation":* Cited in Homola, "Is the Chiropractic Subluxation Theory a Threat to Public Health?"

300: *"use of vaccines":* "American Chiropractic Association Policies on Public Health and Related Matters," 43; can be viewed on the Web at www.amerchiro.org/pdf/2002_aca_policies.pdf; "Canadian Chiropractic Association. Policy Manual," motion 2139 (Toronto: Canadian Chiropractic Association, 1993).

300: *"One small survey of attitudes":* Reported in F. Colley and M. Haas, "Attitudes on Immunization: A Survey of American Chiropractors," *Journal of Manipulative and Physiological Therapeutics* 17 (1994): 584–90.

300: *"A larger study found":* Reported in Anne C. C. Lee, Dawn H. Li, and Kathi J. Kemper, "Chiropractic Care for Children," *Archives of Pediatric and*

Adolescent Medicine 154 (2000): 401–7; can be viewed on the Web at archpedi.ama-assn.org/cgi/content/abstract/154/4/401.

301: *"In a 2002 survey":* Reported in Susan M. Yussman, Peggy Auinger, Michael Weitzman, and Sheryl A Ryan, "Complementary and Alternative Medicine Use in Children and Adolescents in the United States," 2002 Pediatric Academic Societies Abstract; can be viewed on the Web at www.aap.org/research/abstracts/02abstract22.htm.

301: *"chronic or recurring illnesses":* Reported in Anju Sikand and Marilyn Laken, "Pediatricians' Experience With and Attitudes Toward Complementary/Alternative Medicine," *Archives of Pediatric and Adolescent Medicine* 152 (November 1998): 11:1059–64; can be viewed on the Web at archpedi.ama-assn.org/cgi/content/abstract/152/11/1059.

301: *"after taking herbal remedies":* See Paula Gardiner and Kathi J. Kemper, "Herbs in Pediatric and Adolescent Medicine," *Pediatrics in Review* 21 (February 2000): 2:44–57.

301: *"In Massachusetts":* Reported in Anne C. C. Lee and Kathi J. Kemper, "Homeopathy and Naturopathy: Practice Characteristics and Pediatric Care," *Archives of Pediatric and Adolescent Medicine* 154 (2000): 1:75–80; can be viewed on the Web at archpedi.ama-assn.org/cgi/content/abstract/154/1/75.

301: *"Rosemary Gladstar":* Rosemary Gladstar, *Herbal Remedies for Children's Health* (Pownal, Vt.: Storey, 1999), 10.

302: *"while Gladstar claims":* Gladstar, *Herbal Remedies for Children's Health,* 11.

302: *"Gladstar examines":* Gladstar, *Herbal Remedies for Children's Health,* 24.

302: *"University of Arizona Medical Center":* See Carla McClain, "Alternatives for Cerebral Palsy Patients," *Arizona Daily Star,* June 18, 2001; can be viewed on the Web at www.azstarnet.com/health/illness/neuro/cp-epil/cp-10618.shtml.

SUBJECT INDEX

Christian
Medical
Association
Resources

Medically reliable ... biblically sound. That's the rock-solid promise of this series offered by Zondervan in partnership with the Christian Medical Association. Each book in this series is not only written by fully credentialed, experienced doctors but is also fully reviewed by an objective board of qualified doctors to ensure its reliability. Because when your health is at stake, you can't settle for anything less than the whole and accurate truth.

Integrating your faith and health can improve your physical well-being and even extend your life, as you gain insights into the interconnection of health and faith—a relationship largely overlooked by secular science. Benefit from the cutting-edge knowledge of respected medical experts as they help you make health care decisions consistent with your beliefs. Their sound biblical analysis of emerging treatments and technologies equips you to protect yourself from seemingly harmless—yet spiritually, ethically, or medically unsound—options and then to make the healthiest choices possible.

Through this series, you can draw from both the knowledge of science and the wisdom of God's Word in addressing your medical ethics decisions and in meeting your health care needs.

Founded in 1931, the Christian Medical Association helps thousands of doctors minister to their patients by imitating the Great Physician, Jesus Christ. Christian Medical Association members provide a Christian voice on medical ethics to policy makers and the media, minister to needy patients on medical missions around the world, evangelize and disciple students on more than 90 percent of the nation's medical school campuses, and provide educational and inspirational resources to the church.

To learn more about Christian Medical Association ministries and resources on health care and ethical issues, browse the website (www.christian medicalassociation.org) or call toll-free at 1-888-231-2637.

"Dear friend, I pray that you may enjoy good health and that all may go well with you, even as your soul is getting along well" (3 John 2).

God's Design for the Highly Healthy Person

Walt Larimore, M.D., with Traci Mullins

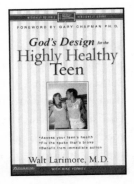

A must-have resource for pursuing wellness, coping with illness, and developing a plan to care for your health needs. Learn how to assess your health, fix the "spoke" that's broke, and benefit from immediate action for improving your life and health.

God's Design for the Highly Healthy Person is like having your very own health mentor to guide you in your total health picture, from treating illness and navigating the health care system to developing a proactive approach to vibrant health.

Softcover: 0-310-26279-8

God's Design for the Highly Healthy Teen

Walt Larimore, M.D., with Mike Yorkey

Good news! An on-call, day or night health consultant for parents—now available for you during those critical (and often scary) teen years. Dr. Walt Larimore is on call, and he's applying his wisdom to your teen's health.

God's Design for the Highly Healthy Teen will help you assess your teen's health, zero in where your teen's health is out of balance, and follow practical, achievable advice that can result in positive changes in your teen's life—and in the process, you'll become a more highly healthy parent.

Softcover: 0-310-24032-8

Alternative Medicine
The Christian Handbook

Dónal O'Mathúna, Ph.D., and
Walt Larimore, M.D.

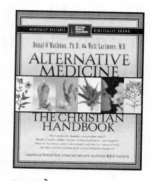

In today's health-conscious culture, options for the care and healing of the body are proliferating like never before. But which ones can you trust?

Alternative Medicine is the first comprehensive guidebook to non-traditional medicine written from a distinctively Christian perspective. Here at last is the detailed and balanced coverage of alternative medicine that you've been looking for. Professor and researcher Dónal O'Mathúna, Ph.D., and national medical authority Walt Larimore, M.D., draw on their extensive knowledge of the Bible and their medical and pharmaceutical expertise to answer the questions about alternative medicine that you most want answered—and others you wouldn't have thought to ask.

This informative resource includes two alphabetical reference sections and a handy cross-reference tool that links specific health problems with various alternative therapies and herbal remedies reviewed in the book. Five categories of alternative medicine are defined and then applied to every therapy and remedy evaluated.

Softcover: 0-310-23584-7

Pick up a copy today at your favorite bookstore!

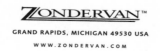

GRAND RAPIDS, MICHIGAN 49530 USA

WWW.ZONDERVAN.COM

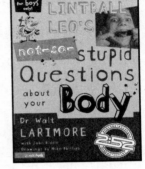
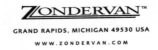

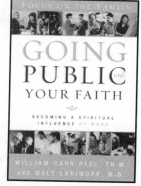
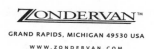

Bryson City Tales

*Stories of a Doctor's First Year
of Practice in the Smoky Mountains*

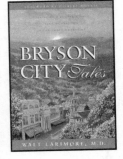

The little mountain hamlet of Bryson City, North Carolina, offers more than dazzling vistas. For Walt Larimore, a young "flatlander" physician setting up his first practice, the town presents its peculiar challenges as well. Sharing the joys, heartaches, frustrations, and rewards of rural mountain medical practice, *Bryson City Tales* is a tender and insightful chronicle of a young man's rite of passage from medical student to family physician. Laughter and adventure await you in these pages, and lessons learned from the strengths, foibles, and simple faith of Bryson City's unforgettable residents.

Softcover: 0-310-25670-4

Bryson City Seasons

*More Tales of a Doctor's Practice
in the Smoky Mountains*

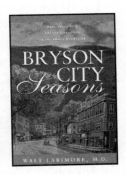

Dr. Walt Larimore whisks you along on a journey through the seasons of another year in Bryson City. On the way you'll encounter crusty mountain men, warmhearted townspeople, peppery medical personalities, and the hallmarks of a more wholesome way of life. Dr. Larimore's vibrant slices of small-town living will capture your imagination and inspire your heart. Lit with love, humor, glowing faith, and the warmth of family and friendships, *Bryson City Seasons* is a celebration of this richly textured miracle called life.

Hardcover: 0-310-25287-3

Pick up a copy at your favorite bookstore today!

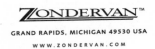

GRAND RAPIDS, MICHIGAN 49530 USA

WWW.ZONDERVAN.COM